A Practical Guide to Pediatric Acupuncture

by the same author

Chinese Medicine for Childhood Anxiety and Depression
A Practical Guide for Practitioners and Parents
Rebecca Avern
Foreword by Elisa Rossi
Illustrated by Sarah Hoyle
ISBN 978 1 78775 781 3
eISBN 978 1 78775 782 0

Acupuncture for Babies, Children and Teenagers
Treating Both the Illness and the Child
Rebecca Avern
Foreword by Julian Scott
Illustrated by Sarah Hoyle
ISBN 978 1 84819 322 2
eISBN 978 0 85701 275 3

Why Do Children Become Ill?
Rebecca Avern
eISBN 978 1 78775 841 4

A Practical Guide to PEDIATRIC ACUPUNCTURE

Rebecca Avern

FOREWORD BY
DR. STEPHEN COWAN MD

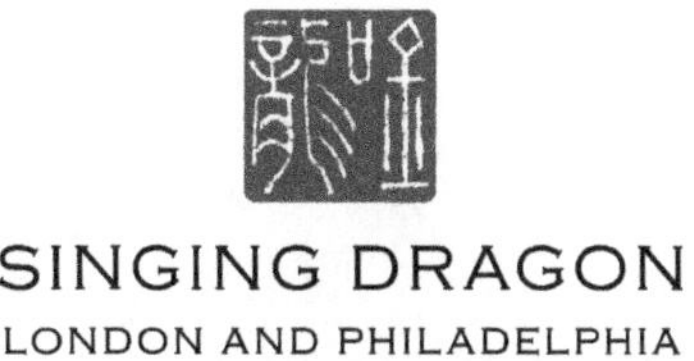

SINGING DRAGON
LONDON AND PHILADELPHIA

First published in Great Britain in 2026 by Singing Dragon,
an imprint of Jessica Kingsley Publishers
Part of John Murray Press

1

Copyright © Rebecca Avern 2026
Illustrations copyright © Sophie Standing 2026
Diagram 4.1 © Shutterstock 2026

Front cover image source: Shutterstock®. The cover image is for illustrative purposes only, and any person featuring is a model.

All rights reserved. No part of this publication may be reproduced, stored in a retrieval system, or transmitted, in any form or by any means without the prior written permission of the publisher, nor be otherwise circulated in any form of binding or cover other than that in which it is published and without a similar condition being imposed on the subsequent purchaser.

A CIP catalogue record for this title is available from the
British Library and the Library of Congress

ISBN 978 1 80501 371 6
eISBN 978 1 80501 372 3

Printed and bound in Great Britain by CPI Group

Jessica Kingsley Publishers' policy is to use papers that are natural, renewable and recyclable products and made from wood grown in sustainable forests. The logging and manufacturing processes are expected to conform to the environmental regulations of the country of origin.

Singing Dragon
Carmelite House
50 Victoria Embankment
London EC4Y 0DZ

www.singingdragon.com

John Murray Press
Part of Hodder & Stoughton Limited
An Hachette UK Company

The authorized representative in the EEA is Hachette Ireland,
8 Castlecourt Centre, Dublin 15, D15 XTP3, Ireland (email: info@hbgi.ie)

This book is dedicated to my husband Peter,
my soulmate and partner in life and love.

Contents

Foreword

医者意也

yīzhě yì yě

Medicine is Intention/Attention

SŪN SĪ MIAO[1*]

"I think of acupuncture as a medicine of the heart." So Rebecca Avern tells us in her wonderful new book, *A Practical Guide to Pediatric Acupuncture*. This heart-based medicine is encapsulated in the seal-script character *yi* 意, which depicts the sounds emanating from the heart. As with every Chinese character, the meaning will depend on the context. *Yi* can be interpreted as intention, attention, idea and/or meaning. Through clinical stories and practical strategies, *A Practical Guide to Pediatric Acupuncture* gives us access to Rebecca's heart, her enthusiasm, her attention to

* Elisa Rossi notes in her book *Shen, Psycho-Emotional Aspects of Chinese Medicine* (2007, Churchill Livingston, pg. 272) that "Medicine is Intention 医者意也" implies that "When one has a patient in front of him, he must use intention for evaluating." As noted in *The Doctor's Intention* (Peking University Third Hospital, Peking University Third School of Clinical Medicine, May 26, 2022) "Medicine is Intention" is a well-known proverb that has a long history in Chinese medicine. It is thought to possibly originate with the famous doctor Guo Yu noted in the *Book of the Later Han Dynasty* by Fan Ye of the Southern Song Dynasty. Sūn Sī Miao of the Tang Dynasty also quoted this in Part 2 of *Appended Formulas Worth a Thousand Nuggets of Gold* Beiji qianjin yaofang 備急千金要方 entitled "On the Great Physician's Sincerity."

detail and her true intention to teach ways to relieve human suffering. It is through this that we as practitioners discover the true meaning of healing.

Rebecca speaks of, "the art of being a pediatric practitioner," a phrase I am deeply drawn to as a practitioner and artist in my own experience working with children. What does it mean to be an artist of medicine? She describes this kind of artistry in healing as a cultivation of "soft skills." Laozi refers to the tremendous power of the soft to overcome the hard, a fundamental skill I have personally experienced in my years of Taichi practice. In the Taichi classics, it states, "the *yi* 意 moves the *qi* 氣,"[2] not the other way around. When instead, the *qi* moves the *yi*, it always runs the risk of being forced and causing tremendous suffering. Children teach us this every day. You can't really force a child to get healthy (nor behave correctly, for that matter). This power of softness is what I think contrasts Chinese medical arts with Western pharmaceutical medicine.

To me, the art of being a skilled pediatric practitioner means being attentive as soon as you walk into a room with a sick child or worried parent. Taking care to observe before jumping to conclusions, allowing time for patterns of relationships to generate meanings that will then be genuine guides to effective treatment. All this is what Sūn Sī Miao meant by, "*yi* 意 must come before treatment *yi* 医." How well we relate to our surroundings is an ecological principle that Chinese medicine has known for thousands of years. Modern research has only now begun to show just how fundamental this kind of "relational health" is in promoting resilience and recovery in children. So much so that it is now a term adopted by the American Academy of Pediatrics as a policy.

I first met Rebecca through her amazing Hub of Pediatric Acupuncture (HOPA) online community. That Hub reflects her Earth nature and healing spirit. Those of us who have been lucky enough to participate in that community are aware of the level of caring and attention she is promoting in the world. Rebecca's emphasis on developing rapport in her relationships with children, parents and practitioners is what makes her a genuine leader in our field.

As described in the great Chinese classics (*Neijing, Nanjing*), the Earth/soil phase traditionally sits in the central position of the great Five Phase cycle. The other four phases (Water, Wood, Fire, Metal) correlate with the four directions and four seasons moving around and through it. It is this central Earth hub that is responsible for making sure the four are related, getting along, harmonizing. Like the Hub that Rebecca created for practitioners, Earth/soil is the ground we stand on, meet and grow in. It is no accident then that the Spleen corresponds with this central position in Chinese medicine and is so fundamental in treating all children. Nor is it coincidence that *yi* 意 is considered the spirit of the Spleen earth. Such caring attention provides the ground from which all nurturing takes place.

The Earth-centered healthcare that Rebecca offers in this book is exactly what the world desperately needs right now. The clinical conditions we are being asked to treat, from dramatic rises in asthma and allergies, to the chronic anxieties, auto-immune diseases, attention deficit hyperactivity disorder (ADHD) and autism (and that's just the conditions that start with the letter "A"!), all share in one fundamental problem: disconnection and alienation. One has only to look at the way we are treating our dear mother Earth to recognize the ecological crises we are facing in the world and within ourselves.

For those of you eager to work with children in your practice, Rebecca's intention/attention will provide invaluable meaning to your development as a clinician. As the Buddha so wisely said, "Attention is our most precious treasure." Rebecca has provided just such a treasure in *A Practical Guide to Pediatric Acupuncture*, which should be on everyone's bookshelf as an invaluable resource and inspiration for years to come.

Dr. Stephen Cowan MD
Year of the Wood/Green Snake 2025

Acknowledgements

Even though at times birthing a book may feel like a solitary process, there are so many people who contribute to its eventual form and content that it feels hard to know where to begin acknowledging them all.

I could not have written this book or, indeed, do most of what I do if it were not for my family. The love of my husband, Peter, and my children, Alathea and Leyla, is a constant source of support, inspiration and nourishment. It's what gets me out of bed in the morning and sustains me when I want to give up. I know that embarking on writing a book does not always make me easy to live with, and their ability to accommodate that is something I both thank and admire them all for.

Peter also, once again, has read every single chapter of this book (twice) and given me his insightful feedback and suggestions that have made it far more readable than it otherwise would have been. He has, once again, given up hours of his own precious time to support me in this project. When I wrote my first book, *Acupuncture for Babies, Children and Teenagers*, Alathea and Leyla were young girls in their first cycle of *jing*. They are now nearing the end of their teen years and getting ready to make their way into the world after school. Every day I love them more, even though every day I would not think that possible. Girls, you are both the most awesome young women, and watching your *jing* unfold and your *shen* manifest has been and continues to be the most phenomenal experience of my life.

I sometimes consider myself to live under a lucky star when it comes to the teachers I have been fortunate enough to learn from over my 25 or so years of practice. Whilst too numerous to mention, those that stand out as having informed my pediatric practice are Julian Scott, the late Giovanni Maciocia, Peter Mole, John and Angie Hicks, the late Alex Tiberi, Thomas Wernicke, Elisa Rossi, Stephen Cowan and Sabine Wilms. There are many, many more whose wisdom I have been able to incorporate into my treatment of children. What I share in this book is underpinned by other writers, teachers and practitioners who have come before me. I truly stand on their shoulders.

I have now been treating young people for 25 years. These children and teenagers have been and continue to be my greatest teachers. Every time I meet a new child in clinic, I learn something new. They also inspire me, make me laugh, impress me, and warm and open my heart, as well as challenging me. This book has really arisen out of my interactions with the huge numbers of little people whom I have treated. I extend my huge gratitude to all of them for allowing me to do my best to help them during a time when life felt tricky.

This is my third book published by Singing Dragon. Once again, I have received support and clarity above and beyond what I could have expected. I thank Claire Wilson, who I have known since I embarked on my first book in 2017 and is always such a huge pleasure to work with. Jenny Edwards has patiently answered all my questions throughout the process. There are many more members of the Singing Dragon team with whom I have not had direct contact but who I know do phenomenal work behind the scenes. A massive thank you also goes to Sophie Standing for coming up with her delightful illustrations, so quickly and so amenably.

Last, but not least, I want to acknowledge all the practitioners of Traditional East Asian Medicines (TEAMs) who have chosen to extend their work to where it is most needed and to work with children. I know it is not easy work, though it is also joyous and wonderful. You are taking your skills to where they are going to have the biggest impact, and it is my deep desire that this book helps support you to continue doing that and to do it more. You are making a difference, even on days when it doesn't feel like it. Thank you.

Introduction

This book is part of my mission in life to encourage, persuade, enthuse and educate practitioners of Traditional East Asian Medicines (TEAMs) to treat more children and teenagers. The mission feels ever more urgent. Day after day, we are confronted by the negative impact that so many aspects of modern life are having on our children. We read devastating statistics that reflect how our changing world is causing ever more suffering in young people. Good physical and mental health seem to be becoming more elusive for more and more of the younger generation. At the same time, children's health services are unable to keep up with demand or simply do not have the tools with which to help.

Yet we do have these tools! In my 25 years of practice, I have seen over and over again how effective, and sometimes even miraculous, our medicine can be in transforming a child's health and potentially therefore changing the trajectory of their life. Whether it's reducing reliance on steroid inhalers, quelling anxiety or banishing adolescent acne, TEAMs are very often the whole or a large part of the solution.

So, why do more children not receive acupuncture? It is my belief that there are two main blocks.

The first is that the majority of TEAMs practitioners leave college having had half a day or a day of training in pediatrics. Some have even been discouraged from thinking about applying our medicine to children. Whilst there are now a good number of books on TEAMs pediatrics in English, and opportunities to study pediatrics at postgraduate level, I have realized that this is not enough. Practitioners are often lacking guidance in the "soft skills" associated with treating children, as well as enough guidance on how to deliver their treatment to children.

Section 1—The Art of Treating Children—is aimed at filling this gap and illustrating many of the "soft skills" needed to work with children. It guides the reader through how to approach communicating and creating therapeutic relationships with young people and their families. It illustrates how a child's ill health does not stand in isolation but is often inextricably linked with family members and family dynamics. As more and more of the children we see have an added layer of sensitivity, there is also a chapter on how to approach the treatment of "atypical" children. I hope that Section 1 will convey the fact that how we communicate with young people and their families is not just something which is additional to our treatment but is a central part of it. I want the reader to know that "the little things" we do or we avoid doing when we treat children are actually "the big things" that can have tremendous impact. I want the reader to feel that our medicine can be transformational for even the most sensitive of children.

The second reason that more children do not receive acupuncture is a lack of understanding amongst both practitioners and parents of how to deliver treatment to children. It is common for people not to be able to get past the idea that children, needles and staying still are not a good combination.

Section 2—The Practicalities of Working with Children—therefore focuses on how to deliver treatment to children. This needs a fundamentally different approach to the treatment of adults. Chapter 7 discusses how to adapt traditional methods of treatment to pediatrics, and Chapter 8 discusses modern methods of treatment. Although I consider myself somewhat of a traditionalist, I am grateful every day for some of the modern innovations which help us to deliver treatment in a way that can be tolerated by the vast majority of children. I include many examples from my practice of how to combine different modalities, giving the reader an insight into the day-to-day realities of pediatric clinical life.

My hope is that this book will feel like a supportive companion to practitioners as they navigate the ins and outs of pediatrics. It is not about theory, and for a thorough grounding in TEAMs pediatric theory I refer you to my earlier work, *Acupuncture for Babies, Children and Teenagers*. This book will not teach you which points to choose or how to treat particular conditions, but it will instill you with confidence that TEAMs really is a medicine suitable for children. Most of all, it is my wish that you will come away from reading this book feeling, "Yes—I want to work with little people."

Working with young people has its challenges but, as the great Sūn Sī Miao famously said, "There is no greater *dao*" than this. I urge you to embrace the challenge and to shout from the rooftops that you, as a practitioner of TEAMs, welcome young people into your practice with open arms and are skilled in an exquisite system of medicine with which to be able to help them.

SECTION 1

THE ART OF TREATING CHILDREN

Chapter 1

The Art of Being a Pediatric Practitioner

There is no Dao among the common people that is greater than the Dao of nurturing the young.

SŪN SĪ MIAO[3]

Over 1400 years ago, the great Sūn Sī Miao recognized the importance of looking after babies and children. He knew that the right care, the right treatment, at the right time and to the right degree would impact a child's health in a positive way for the rest of their life. In his seminal text *Essential Formulas to Prepare for Emergencies, Worth a Thousand in Gold* (*Bèijí Qiānjīn Yàofāng*), he laid out herbal formulas and acupuncture treatments for common childhood conditions and expounded his views on the type of care babies needed.

We acupuncturists and TEAMs practitioners are now fortunate enough to have relatively easy access to a wealth of texts on the theory of TEAMs pediatrics. In order to treat children effectively, it is essential to profoundly understand this theory and be able to apply it to the treatment of children.

Sūn Sī Miao also talked about the *dao* of treating children, which is so much more than simply putting theory into practice. If we are to be successful pediatric practitioners, we need to find our way and cultivate our art. This is the real work. This is what distinguishes someone who heals children from someone who merely treats children.

Imagine the following (not uncommon) scenario. A mother comes to your clinic with her six-month-old baby who is posseting milk after every feed. She is exhausted and distressed. She feels she may be "doing something wrong" and that her baby is not thriving. You know that posseting can be due to weak or cold Stomach *qi* which fails to descend properly. You could help this mother and baby significantly by choosing appropriate points and techniques to rectify the imbalance.

In addition, you might choose to allow the mother time to share with you (if she chooses) how she is feeling. You might be still and present while she sheds tears of guilt that the birth did not go as she had hoped. You might point out to her how well her baby is, despite the posseting. You might carry out your treatment in a sensitive way that the baby tolerates well. You might explain to the mother what you are doing and why. You might let her know that you are here to help if problems arise in the future.

This level of care and attention is what will distinguish you as what Sūn Sī Miao called a "Great Doctor"[4] (Wilms' translation of the term *dà yī*). It will mean you get better results and help many children more profoundly. Importantly, it will also mean *you* will feel nourished by your work and will be able to sustain it over a longer period of time.

So let's take a deeper look at creating *your* personalized, individual and unique *dao* of nurturing the young.

The art of pediatrics through a Five Phase lens

Using the lens of the Five Phases *wu xing* is a great way of highlighting the qualities we need to bring to our pediatric practice. As the Five Phases sit differently in all of us, you will have some of these qualities in abundance, whilst others may be more difficult to summon. The key is to play to your strengths and recognize your weaknesses. For example, I have an abundance of Earthy, mothering *qi*, so the little people who come to my clinic feel they get a lot of nurture and mother love. On the flip side, my Earth can get a bit "boggy" at times, which means my vibe can be heavy. So sometimes I need to work on keeping light and joyful. My colleague Tom, on the other hand, tends to hang out in his Fire. His treatments are all fun and games and he manages to get every child laughing without breaking a sweat. So Tom and I bring very different qualities to our practice, but the crucial thing is we each bring who we are. We cultivate our strengths to make sure we are healing kids, not only treating them.

In the 1950s, there was a report in *The Lancet* from an eminent physician called Dr. Balint. He wrote about a discussion he'd had with colleagues at the Tavistock Clinic concerning their most commonly prescribed drugs. He described how they soon realized that the most frequently prescribed drug was in fact the doctor himself! Over the following decades, this led to doctors being trained to recognize the profound implications of how they conduct their interactions and build relationships with their patients. Remember, to some degree, you *are* your medicine. Or at the very least, how you deliver your medicine is a large part of the medicine itself.

Fire

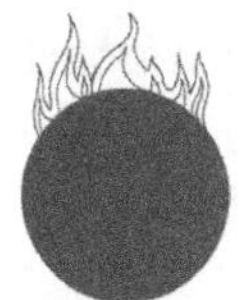

The spirit of Fire is the *shen*. The *shen* enables us to be fully in the present moment and have a general awareness of the situation.

Other Fire qualities can greatly enhance the way we practice.

Uniqueness

Winnie the Pooh, an almost unrivalled source of wisdom, said that, "The things that make me different are the things that make me, me."[5] He could have been speaking of the *shen* of the Heart, which Larre and Rochat de la Vallée explained is, "that by which a given being is unlike any other; that which makes an individual an individual and more than a person."[6]

Babies, children and teenagers have very well-tuned "in-authenticity detectors." The greatest gift you can give them is your unique self. It will engender better connection and also model to them that they can be themselves when they are with you.

It would, of course, be inappropriate to bring into our clinics every aspect of our beings. The children we work with do not need to be exposed to the worry, sadness or anger that might be plaguing us on a particular day. They key point is that the persona we embody as we do our work must resonate with our true nature, which is contained in our *jing* and manifested by the *shen*.

Connection and communication

The organs of the Fire phase enable us to have heart-to-heart connection with others. When I interact with you, the *shen* of my Heart is relating to the *shen* of your Heart—not only through the words we speak but via all sorts of non-verbal signals too. If the *shen* is securely and peacefully housed in my Heart and if my Pericardium (the Heart Protector) is appropriately open, it allows for the possibility of deep connection. This is a prerequisite for a successful therapeutic relationship.

The more healthy the Fire organs are, the more we can create the possibility of profound, therapeutic connection. Of course, interaction is dependent on both parties. But as the practitioner and the adult, our job is to lead the way and create the best circumstances possible.

Once we have created a deep connection with the young people we see and their parents, it allows for proper communication. Good communication is at the heart of what we do. We may be carrying out wonderful treatments, but unless we communicate in a way and to a degree that fits the needs of the child and their family, we are limiting the scope of what we can achieve.

Joy

Ling Shu Chapter 8 tells us of the relationship between Fire and the emotion of joy:

> The Heart is in control of the blood vessels and the spirit resides in the blood vessels. A hollowness of the energy in the Heart will cause the emotion of sadness; a solidness of the energy in the Heart will cause incessant laughter.[7]

The two characters for joy (*xi* and *le*) convey the idea of the ability of people to sing, make music, enjoy themselves and have a good time. Joyfulness is healing. Moreover, the vast majority of young people cannot resist some fun. Mary Poppins sang that, "a spoonful of sugar helps the medicine go down."[8] Equally, a small dose of fun and laughter helps the treatment "go down."

I am not talking here about forced or false joy or laughter. The important thing is to be open to moments of spontaneous humor and fun. Young children especially are masters of seeing the funny side of things. Allowing the flames of our Fire to respond and be lifted by this helps to create a lightness during our treatment sessions, which is beneficial for everyone.

> Four-year-old Leo thought it was really funny to grab one of the silicone cups I was using on his stomach and put it on my face. I had a choice in that moment. I could either get a bit irritated, as it was disrupting the flow of my treatment, or I could incorporate his little game *into the flow* of my treatment, whilst putting a few boundaries in place about what was acceptable (no cups on my eyes please!). By choosing the latter response, I was able to maintain the flow and keep Leo on board with the treatment. Furthermore, through having some fun, my connection with Leo deepened and he left the session with a felt experience of having had a good time.

Enthusiasm

Enthusiasm is contagious. When you connect with a love of your work, parents and children will notice that. I have a dental hygienist who is in love with teeth! It is quite obvious that she finds teeth totally fascinating. It makes me want to go and see her, as I know she will look after my teeth, rather than someone else who is just going through the motions. It is when you feel passionate that you bring your heart into your work; you excel at it and people want to come and see you.

Emotional warmth

In the Worsley Five Phase tradition, a question often asked is: "What does a person of each element type most need?" The answer to the question of what a Fire type most needs is emotional warmth. Whatever the element type, many children respond to warmth. When a practitioner is able to act with genuine warmth to a child, it will make the child feel accepted and comfortable, and safe. Of course, there are some children for whom too intense a display of warmth may feel overwhelming. However, generally speaking, children love warmth and do not respond well to emotional coldness.

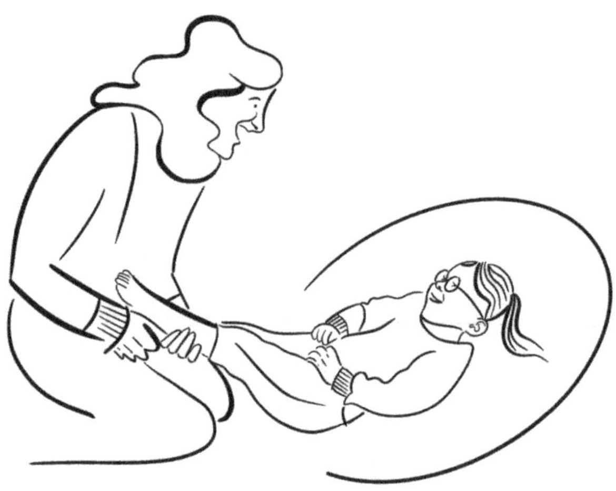

Metal

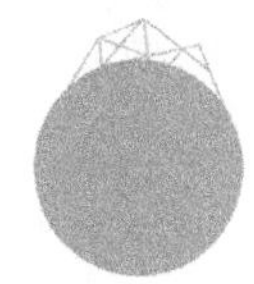

The spirit of Metal is the *po*. The *po* allows us to tune in to our instincts and to "pick up the vibes" as to what is going on.

Other Metal qualities can greatly enhance the way we practice.

Inspiration

The Metal phase is resonant with breathing in, not only in the physical sphere but also in the spiritual one. The *yin* organ of Metal, the Lung, is said to be, "The Receiver of qi from the Heavens."[9] When our Lung *qi* is strong, we feel connected to the "heavenly *qi*," meaning our lives will have a sense of quality and higher purpose. As practitioners, we need to stay connected to our feelings of inspiration in relation to the extraordinary power of our medicine. The moment we lose that sense of awe and become immune to its magic, we lose potency as a healer. The little people who come to see us, with their sharp emotional antennae, will pick up on our feelings towards the medicine we practice. Nobody will feel safe and hopeful in the hands of someone who is bored and disconnected from the spirit of their work.

Righteousness

Righteousness, or having a clear sense of right and wrong, stems from the Metal phase. This quality is essential in clinic to guide us when the situation is murky and the way through not clear. Righteousness is akin to having a strong moral compass. It leads us, for example, to be open with a parent when we know we cannot help their child. It means we will risk the disapproval of a parent when it feels right to support their teenager's perspective over theirs. It ensures we acknowledge and apologize for a wrong turn we have taken in treatment instead of covering it up. Having a strong degree of righteousness ensures that we remain an ethical practitioner.

Order and precision

Su Wen Chapter 8 says:

> The Lung holds the office of minister and chancellor. The regulation of the life-giving network stems from it.[10]

The Lung, and specifically its spirit the *po* (the corporeal soul), helps to bring about regulation in the body so that the right thing happens at the right time and there is a sense of rhythm to the bodily processes. If we carry this quality to the external world, on a practical level, running a successful pediatric clinic requires some degree of order and organization. Managing several young people in your room at one time (siblings often come in tow), some of whom may be keen on exploring everything they see, requires you to approach your work in a structured and orderly manner. Furthermore, most children will not feel safe or contained in a chaotic environment.

The importance of precision as an acupuncturist is self-evident. Not only do we need to be precise with our needles, but we also need to be precision-focused in every aspect of our treatments. Observing every component of a child's being, and being precise in our words and our actions, enhances the power of our treatments.

Children who come to see us are not islands. They are part of an entire system made up of their immediate family, extended family, community and friends. They may come into the world carrying patterns from previous generations. They often arrive with complex feelings regarding their health struggles. Their parent may be anxious or even despairing. All of this means that we, the practitioner, may feel somewhat bombarded with information and emotions. A quality of the Metal phase is to be able to "cut through" to what is important with precision.

Twelve-year-old Sonia came to see me, with both her parents and her brother, after several years of quite brutal cancer treatment. Sonia was now in remission. She and her family had patently been through years of emotional agony and physical endurance. They told me in detail about Sonia's medical journey over the last six years from the day she was diagnosed with cancer. They all cried at different times during the session. Sonia was currently suffering several debilitating symptoms as a result of her cancer treatment. The atmosphere was buzzing with huge amounts of complex information as well as intense and conflicting emotions from all four family members. This was a time when I needed to use the powers of Metal to cut through to what was important. Sonia told me that what she most wanted was simply to feel joyful again. I was able to put everything else that had been communicated in the session to one side and direct my treatment at what would most help Sonia in that moment.

Earth

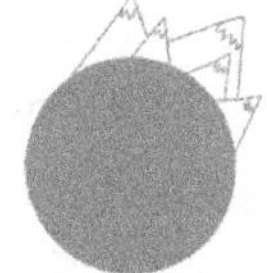

The spirit of Earth is the *yi*. The *yi* allows us to digest, process and integrate all the information we receive during a session.

Other Earth qualities can greatly enhance the way we practice.

Mother love

The Earth phase is the mother and the center from which nourishment comes. Larre and Rochat de la Vallée describe the character *tu di* as the soil on which plants grow but also the ability of the earth to be like a mother.[11] The desire to look after and care for people is an obvious attribute for a practitioner, especially one who wants to work with children. Young children can rarely get too much of it; older children and teenagers may accept it more easily from someone who is not their actual parent. Cultivating a grounded, centered quality will mean that children feel safe and looked after in your presence.

Parents will appreciate it too. The responsibility of parenting can drain the organs of the Earth phase. I often invite the parent who brings their child for treatment to take some time out while I care for their child during the session. This small act can provide a parent with a break from the relentlessness of parenting and the feeling that it is all down to them.

Empathy

In the Worsley Five Phase tradition, the "emotion" associated with the Earth phase is sympathy. I prefer to talk of empathy. There are important differences between the two. Empathy is done *with* somebody rather than *to* somebody. It is an attempt to understand another's point of view in all its complexity rather than to pity or feel sorry for somebody. A person on the receiving end of empathy will feel validated and cared for, not patronized. This is the quality that healthy Earth organs enable us to have and which potentiates so much healing.

A little word of warning, however. As practitioners, we should strive to open ourselves up to being fully empathic when we are with the young people in our clinics who need help. Yet if we find ourselves spending lots of time outside of clinic thinking about them, or notice we have a slightly desperate need to "get them better," we need to be mindful. Both of these things may be a sign that our Earth has lost its center. This tends to get in the way of healing and also means we may end up burnt out and resentful, having given too much of ourselves.

Yi

We mentioned the *yi* above but the *yi* is so important in our discussion of practicing medicine that it deserves further mention.

Yi is often translated as intention. In order to practice medicine well, we must employ our *yi*. The character for *yi* includes both the heart radical and a radical for a musical note. Wilms suggests translating this as "heart-sounding."[12] In *Ling Shu* Chapter 8, we read that, "when the heart applies itself, we speak of Intent (*yi*)."[13] So, although *yi* is often associated with intellect and thinking, it also encompasses the heart. It beautifully encapsulates the idea that to practice medicine well involves both the mind and the heart working together.

We must focus our *yi* in two directions. First, our *yi* helps us to penetrate and understand the subtleties and profundity of the clinical situation. Second, our *yi* helps us to carry out the appropriate treatment in a focused and effective way.

As Sūn Sī Miao implores, when you treat, "your *shen* should be as fine as autumn down, with your *yi* fixed only on the patient."[14]

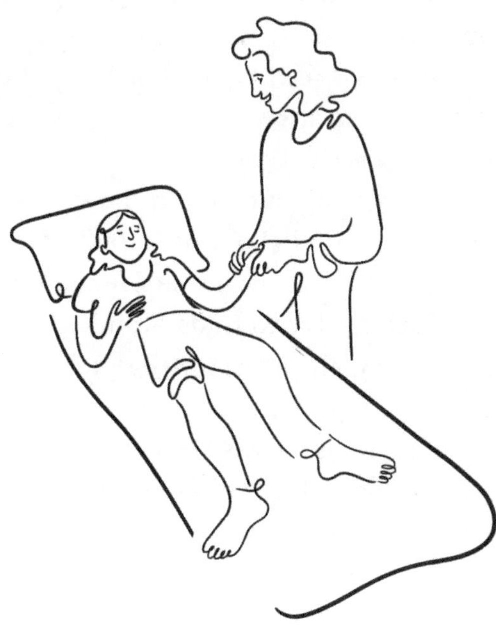

Wood

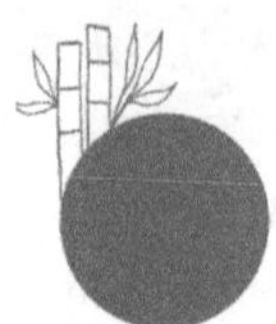

The spirit of Wood is the *hun*. The *hun* allows us to imagine and envision what healing would look like in a particular child and devise a plan to get them there.

Other Wood qualities can greatly enhance the way we practice.

Compassion

The virtue of the Wood phase is compassion (*ren*). As Bob Dylan sang, "Remember when you're out there trying to heal the sick, that you must always first forgive them."[15] There is an unhelpful notion that, as healers, we naturally feel compassion towards all those we work with, especially when they are children. Most practitioners, when being entirely honest, would probably admit that it is just not that easy. Some of the young people and their parents who arrive in our clinics will trigger less-than-noble feelings in us. It is the organs of the Wood phase that enable us to transform irritation, frustration or anger into compassion. True healing will not take place without it.

This, of course, begs the question of how we go about developing compassion. I find the most effective way of doing this is by being curious. If I find myself feeling irritated by a behavior or a narrative, I try to understand what is behind it rather than allowing myself to react with rigidity. Once I understand it more, my feeling response changes and I can usually summon my compassion towards the person. Fundamentally, compassion is to recognize our shared humanity and to act in the best interests of another rather than ourselves. Sūn Sī Miao encapsulated the idea of compassion beautifully when he said, "When you witness the pain and suffering of others, you must act as if they were your own and open your heart deeply to their misery."[16]

> I found myself getting irritated with ten-year-old Nial. He was always messing around and using endless delay tactics, and was antagonistic towards me and his mum. Early on in one session, Nial said, "Acupuncture is so weird and it's obviously not going to help me anyway." I noticed myself feeling irritated but took a deep breath and was able to change my response. Instead of interpreting Nial's words as a criticism or dismissal, I heard them this time as an expression of confusion and not knowing. I started pointing out to Nial certain things on my acupuncture charts and talked to him about what I was doing and why I was doing it. Nial is now one of acupuncture's greatest fans, and our relationship has completely changed.

Assertion

When the organs of the Wood phase are balanced, we can excel at being assertive without being bossy. This is important when working with children. On the one hand, parents need to feel we have appropriate authority if they are to entrust their child's care to us. On the other hand, many young people will not respond well to an overbearing authority. We need to be in charge without that being obvious or overt. We are aiming for an appropriate assertiveness. Think back to your school days. You can probably remember a teacher with whom nobody would muck around and who, without shouting, commanded the respect of even the most disruptive members of the class. We should aim to be a practitioner version of that teacher and have a quiet authority to which children usually respond well.

Planning and strategizing

Su Wen Chapter 8 tells us that, "The Liver holds the office of general of the armed forces. Assessment of circumstances and conception of plans stem from it."[17] Once we have made our diagnosis, we should have a plan in terms of a treatment strategy. Rather than aimlessly moving from one thing that feels like a good idea at the time to another, the organs of the Wood phase allow us to create an insightful vision of how to heal a child over a period of time. This Liver's paired organ, the Gallbladder, then helps us to make good decisions about how to put that plan into practice.

Of course, as we implement our plan, we need to employ huge amounts of flexibility. This really is at the heart of the art of pediatric acupuncture. To be able to keep sight of the end goal, whilst at the same time finding a way of getting there which is well tolerated by the child, is a skill which requires the *qi* of our Liver and Gallbladder to be coursing smoothly.

Water

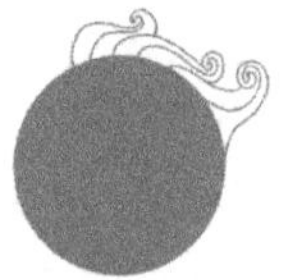

The spirit of Water is the *zhi*. The *zhi* allows us to hold on to our intention over time, to persist and endure despite challenges.

Other Water qualities can greatly enhance the way we practice.

Perseverance furthers

The spirit of Water deserves further mention. The character for *zhi* conveys the idea of being able to persevere towards one's goals without being deflected. It is often translated as "drive" or "willpower" but is perhaps more aptly understood as the power of perseverance or determination.

When working with children, there are times when we need perseverance to be able to carry out and complete the treatment we know the child needs. A young child may be bored or hyperactive or more interested in playing with your toys. We need to persist in keeping them engaged while we treat them. This requires the pediatric practitioner to dig deep and have the conviction to complete the treatment, and having a strong *zhi* will enable them to do this.

Although in many cases children respond to treatment more quickly than adults, as a pediatric practitioner, you will have challenging cases come through your door. Some children you see will be extremely ill or will have an inordinate amount of stress in their lives. It can sometimes feel as if we are trying to swim against the tide. It's easy to become disheartened when we don't get immediate results. Having a strong *zhi* will enable us to persevere when that is what is needed.

There are also times when you might feel the situation is on the verge of being slightly out of control. Maybe there are a couple of bored and feuding siblings in the room or the level of hyperactivity in a child has become extreme. During these times, it is essential to hold your nerve and persevere.

Calm and serenity

Rudyard Kipling's famous line, "If you can keep your calm when all about you are losing theirs',[18] could have been written for someone who works with children! One of the things I love about pediatric practice is the degree of liveliness, variety and intensity that being around young people brings. However, as practitioners, it is helpful for us to provide a counterbalance to this by summoning our inner stillness. I strive to create a space of serenity and peace in my clinic, where young people and their parents can find some respite from their busy lives.

In a similar vein, harnessing the still, deep quality of Water provides reassurance and helps to allay the inevitable anxiety that comes with being around poorly children and their parents. We need to project a confident and solid aura. Simply being a steady, safe presence allows a young person and their parent to feel held and is a prerequisite for healing to begin.

I feel that Sūn Sī Miao was alluding to this quality of the Water phase when he said:

> This is how you embody a Great Doctor: You want to obtain a spirit that is clear like settled water and inward-looking, present

yourself to others with gravitas and as being in a state of bountiful abundance, and as neither too glorious nor too obscure.[19]

One patient comes to mind where the quality of my *zhi* was put to the test. Nine-year-old Jack had a complex urinary condition that had left doctors flummoxed. He was also on the autism spectrum and was initially reticent to allow me to try any treatment modality. So there was a double challenge of a difficult diagnosis and difficulty implementing treatment. During the course of treatment, I modified my diagnosis several times and had to consistently think "outside the box" as to how I could deliver Jack's treatment in a way he tolerated. He, his parents and I had to summon our will during times we could have easily given up. In the end, we got there. Jack tolerated his treatment, and his urinary symptoms improved.

Flow

I give my best treatments when I am in the flow. It is hard to describe what this really means but we probably all know how it feels. There is a feeling of being in sync and in tune with the young person we are treating and a fluency to how we carry out the treatment. This ability to flow comes from the organs of the Water phase. When balanced, we find we lack hesitancy and we act but we don't "react." Everything seems easy in this state, and we can flow through a busy day feeling that we are doing good work without too much struggle. It is not realistic to expect to *always* be in a flow state. Nevertheless, the more we experience it, the more frequently achievable it becomes.

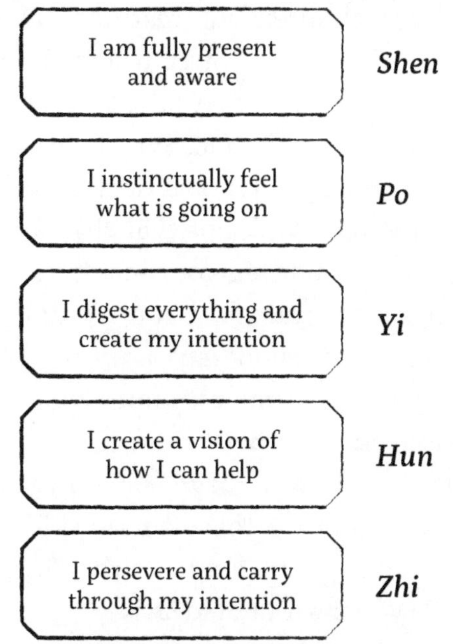

DIAGRAM 1.1 EMPLOYING THE FIVE SPIRITS IN OUR APPROACH TO TREATMENT

Summary

Western medicine places little value on the qualities described above. Its diagnostic methods are largely technological instruments, lab tests and objective number crunching. While there may be nods here and there to the importance of bedside manner, there is little recognition of how these seemingly small yet fundamentally essential attributes transform medical care. As society has come to devalue them, so can we, as practitioners, sometimes doubt their vital importance.

As practitioners, we all have different strengths and weaknesses. The children we see will all need something different from us too. We should try to recognize the emotional qualities described above that we have in abundance and identify the ones we need to work harder to muster. We need to be authentic at the same time as trying to give each individual child what they need.

When working with children, our treatments tend to be minimal and do not take much time. I often hear colleagues say they come out of a session feeling as if they have barely done anything. This feeling may come from the fact that so much of what we do is not obvious or concrete. When a doctor takes someone's temperature, nobody has any doubt that they are performing a task. Yet being present, honing your instinct, focusing your intention, speaking in a certain way, summoning compassion, actively listening or compassionately inquiring are all equally valid forms of "doing." I urge you to remind yourself every day that these Five Phase qualities that you bring to your practice are just as valuable as your skills in diagnosis or needle technique. Indeed, it is through crafting these subtle skills throughout years of practice that we come closer to the kind of "medical virtuosity"* towards which we should strive.

* "Medical virtuosity" is one possible translation of the term *dé* 德 which Wilms translates as "virtue-power" and which Sūn Sī Miao discussed at great length in his two essays "On the Professional Practice of the Great Doctor" and "On the Sublime Sincerity of the Great Doctor," which constitute the first two chapters of his *Essential Formulas to Prepare for Emergencies, Worth a Thousand in Gold.*

CHAPTER 2

The Art of Creating a Therapeutic Relationship with Children

If there is one particular aspect of pediatric practice that sets it apart from treating adults, it is the need to engage children in their treatment. When an adult comes for acupuncture, they have made the decision to do so themselves. When a child comes, the idea has usually originated in the parent. So, from the outset, there is work to be done to convey to the child that you are kind, your aim is to help relieve their suffering and that you will treat them like a human being. This may sound strange. You may be thinking, "Of course everyone treats children as if they are human beings." I don't believe this to be the case. Many children experience and expect to be talked over, ignored, invalidated and coerced. This is really the most basic and fundamental level of welcoming a child to your clinic.

After this, the work of creating rapport begins.

Rapport

What is rapport?

A Dictionary of Psychology, by Oxford University Press, defines rapport as, "a sympathetic or harmonious relationship or state of mutual understanding."[20] In common parlance, we might say that one person "has great rapport" with another, meaning that they "get each other." To have rapport with another person means that you will generally feel relaxed in their company, able to be yourself and that you are trusted and trusting. When there is rapport, there is flow and ease.

There are several characters which reveal the Chinese way of thinking about human relationships, which are, of course, at the heart of medical practice. Studying these characters can help us to understand more deeply the concept of rapport and how to go about creating it. The first is *shu*, which translates as "benevolent, merciful, to pardon."[21] The character is made up of the radical "heart" *xin* and "feeling similar" *ru*. It conveys the idea of empathy and understanding. The second is *zhong*. This character is made up of the radical "center" *zhong* and (again) "heart" *xin*. It conveys the idea of integrity and of heart connection being at the center of any relationship. Third, the character *cheng*, which translates as "authentic, sincere."[22]

So we have some key qualities which we should strive to embody in order to achieve rapport with the little people who come to us for help:

- Benevolence
- Empathy
- Integrity
- Heart connection
- Authenticity.

Reasons for rapport

The relationship is where the healing happens

It is hard to emphasize just how important the relationship between practitioner and patient is in the therapeutic encounter and how much it influences the outcome of treatment. Our needles and our other methods are so incredibly powerful, but when we use them in the context of a healing relationship, they take on superpowers!

I think of acupuncture as a medicine of the heart. Yes, we can resolve damp, move *qi*, clear heat, nourish *yin* etc., etc., but fundamentally, we are creating a relationship within which healing can happen. When a young person feels seen, when we create a space for them to reveal their true nature, when we spark a connection, we are setting the scene for and providing a backdrop against which change begins.

In many of the young people who come to my clinic, I sense a degree of them "holding it together." Life is busy and fast-paced, families are strained and school can be tough. If we can create a space where a child steps outside of this, they can take some deep breaths and their *qi* starts flowing. This provides the perfect springboard from which they can start feeling better, and their symptoms begin to abate.

Rapport enables us to carry out treatment

Confucius wrote:

> If a man is brusque in his movements, others will not cooperate. If he is agitated in his words, they awaken no echo in others. If he asks for something without having first established relations, it will not be given to him.[23]

Confucius's words bring us perfectly to the second reason why rapport is so very important when treating young people. Put simply, if we do not have rapport with a child, they will not let us treat them. Most children who come to see us do not have previous experience of acupuncture and related techniques. A lot of what we do is unfamiliar to them. The idea of needles is, for many children, unnerving or even frightening. We may have made a brilliant diagnosis, have chosen the most appropriate points and techniques to rectify the imbalance. Yet unless we have rapport with the child, our hands will be tied, as there will be very little we can do.

Seven steps to creating rapport

1. Being present

Children have strong antennae for what is going on in those around them. They are impacted by the moods of others. If you are not fully present, they will know. The first step to good rapport is to be fully in the room with the child. The things that prevent us from being fully in the room are usually a preoccupation with the "stuff of life" and stuck emotions.

Each practitioner needs to find a method for emptying their heart and stilling their mind that works for them. What works well for me is taking my dog out for a brisk walk before I start work or doing some yoga. For you, it might be meditating, doing some *qi gong* or playing the piano. It really does not matter what your method is as long as it is effective. It needs to be something which enables you to separate from what does not belong in the moment and leave your mental and emotional preoccupations behind. Sūn Sī Miao wrote:

> Under all circumstances, when you treat disease as a Great Doctor, you must calm your spirit and nail down your will, you must be free of wants and desires, and you must first develop a heart full of great loving-kindness and empathy.[24]

2. Starting with the person not the symptoms

The second step to creating good rapport is to start off your relationship with the young person by focusing on them rather than their symptoms. We want to find out *who* the young person is before we explore *how* the young person is. We want to find out what matters to them before we explore what the matter is. Your primary focus should be trying to get a sense of who this child is in their essence.

The types of questions we might begin with, and which need to be adapted according to age, are:

- I would love to know a little bit about you—what are your favorite things to do?
- I know that you are here with Mum—tell me about some other people in your life.
- I know you are eight, so I am guessing you are in 3rd Grade (Year 4 in the UK) at school. How is 3rd Grade going for you? Can you tell me some of the things you like and don't like about school?

3. Advance and retreat

As you make contact with a child, be sensitive to how they receive it. If their eyes, breathing and body language indicate they like it and are open, you can keep going. If they look away, tense up or lean back, then retreat and change your line of questioning or turn your attention to the parent. Think about how you would approach a nervous puppy. You would probably reach your hand out first before taking small, tentative steps towards them so as not to scare them. Once your hand had made contact with them, you might move the rest of your body closer. Energetically, it is a similar approach with a child. Advance and retreat, advance and retreat. Be focused on everything their body, eyes and words are telling you and let them show you what feels OK for them and what does not. For some children, even making direct eye contact is too much at the start. Put what is socially normal and expected to one side and respond to the child in front of you.

I was working with a 15-year-old boy who was feeling extremely low in mood—to the extent he was struggling to function day to day. In our first session, I asked him about what was going on for him around the time his mood dropped. In this moment, he changed. His eyes dropped downwards, his voice became clipped and he said he didn't know. I had a strong feeling he did in fact know, but he did not yet feel able to share whatever it was. In our second session, I said to him, "I had the feeling it was difficult for you when I asked you about what was going on around the time you began struggling with your mood. I'd love to explore that with you more, but at your pace and only if that feels OK for you. Would that be alright?" He replied that he didn't know if he could talk about it but he would try, and I reassured him that it was absolutely fine to go at his pace. This is an example of the "advance and retreat" approach, where we are led by the signals the young person is giving us.

4. Meeting the needs of the situation

The famous Daoist concept of *wu wei*, often erroneously understood as meaning "non-action," is better understood as, "acting in a way the situation is calling for." Practicing *wu wei* is an art that is honed over time. It is, however, crucial for developing and maintaining rapport with all the young people we work with.

Most practitioners have a way they like to do things and a framework they generally follow in clinic. This may be greeting the family in the waiting room, sitting everybody down to chat about what has happened since the last treatment and then performing the treatment on the child. Whilst this may work well in most situations, there may be times when sticking to this familiar pattern does not meet the needs of the moment.

The best way to illustrate this is to give you some examples from my own clinic. One boy I treat has selective mutism. What works for him is to give him a warm and friendly greeting but to not ask him any questions at all and to get him straight onto the treatment table. His dad always sends me an update via email on the day of the treatment. A teenage girl I have been working with for some time *really* values talking. Sometimes, our entire session is taken up with her talking and me listening. When I first began treating her, she was extremely closed and barely spoke at all. Now that she has found her voice, and her trust in me, there are times when the best way to meet the needs of the moment is to allow her to spend our whole appointment time talking. Another example comes to mind of a boy who likes to have his treatment first and talk afterwards or, more accurately, during. Once the needles are in and his *qi* starts flowing, it is easier for him to let me know how he is feeling.

Employing *wu wei* relies on the practitioner being present, tuned in and aware of the atmosphere. It requires them to be in complete harmony with the young person, as if patient and practitioner were energetically doing a dance together.

In the *Great Compendium of Acupuncture and Moxibustion* (*Zhenjiu Dacheng*), we read:

> In the mind of the physician there should be no desires, only a receptive and accepting attitude, then the mind can become *shen*. The mind of the physician and the mind of the patient should be level, in harmony...[25]

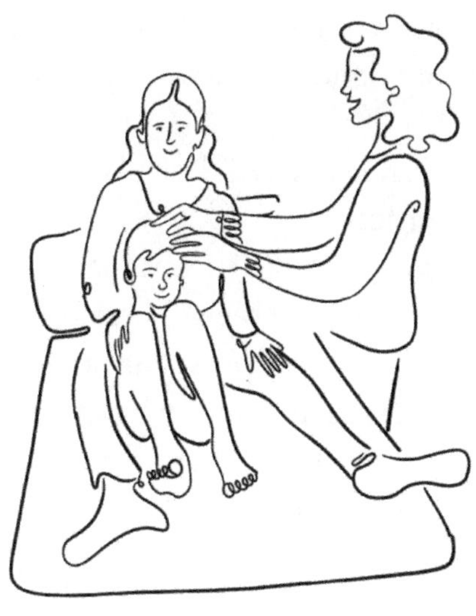

5. Active listening

Sadly, in a world with so much noise, the art of good listening seems to be fading. When we listen well, we allow ourselves to be changed by another person. This means that what we hear moves us away from a preconceived notion of what is and closer to what *really* is. The key to active listening is to listen to understand rather than listen to reply. I find this is especially important to remember when working with teenagers. Really good-quality, active listening is a prerequisite for good rapport. When you listen actively to the young person you are working with, you give them the gift of showing them that they matter and their voice counts. Nobody feels good in a relationship in which they feel there is no space for them.

Listening, however, is not just a function of the ears. A good practitioner listens with their whole being. As Chuang Tzu described:

> The hearing that is only in the ears is one thing. The hearing of the understanding is another. But the hearing of the spirit is not limited to any one faculty, to the ear, or to the mind. Hence it demands the emptiness of all the faculties. And when the faculties are empty, then the whole being listens. There is then a direct grasp of what is right there before you that can never be heard with the ear or understood with the mind."[26]

6. Understanding that every child needs something a little different

One of the reasons it is tricky to write a "script" for how to gain rapport is that every child you see will need something slightly different. The age of the young person is obviously a differentiating factor but so too is their emotional nature. Once again, our Five Phase model is a helpful lens through which to understand what different children need.

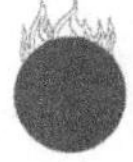

Fire child: Needs warmth, overtly expressed affection and a little dose of fun.

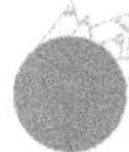

Earth child: Needs nurture, to feel deeply cared for and to be understood and held.

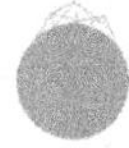

Metal child: Needs an exceedingly gentle "advance," orderliness and to feel valued.

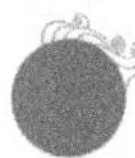

Water child: Needs calm, solidity, reassurance and time to feel their way into your space.

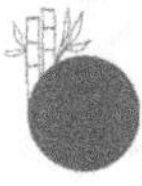

Wood child: Needs firm and clear boundaries, directness and impartiality.

Of course, a child will need different things from you at different times. Sometimes, it's easy to know what a child needs from you but sometimes it is not. When I am struggling to connect with a child, I find it helpful to stand back and ask myself, "How do they need me to be different from how I am being?" My belief is that there is *always* a way to connect, and we just have to keep searching until we find it.

I had seen 14-year-old Zoe for four sessions but just didn't feel I had developed good rapport with her yet. She was quiet and withdrawn and generally answered my questions with as few words as possible. After one particular session, I reflected on what was going on and how I felt with Zoe. I realized that I always came away with the feeling that I was desperately trying to draw her out and that it was hard work. If it was hard work for me, it probably felt like hard work for Zoe too—having to think of answers to all my questions. The next session I decided to suggest to Zoe that she got straight up onto the treatment table rather than sitting opposite me in a chair for a chat. I only asked her one question—was there anything she wanted to share with me today about her week? After a few minutes, Zoe just spontaneously began talking and barely drew breath. She was simply a young person who needed to get to things in her own time and not feel pressured. I still see Zoe to this day, and it still works beautifully if I refrain from talking and let her come to it in her own time!

7. Care and compassion

To say that we should deeply care for and have compassion towards our patients might sound obvious. Most of us have chosen this profession because we want to help reduce suffering. Yet care and compassion are not qualities that simply "are"; they are qualities that need to be practiced. Although in this context they are nouns, we should think of them as verbs.

There are numerous small ways to convey to our young clients that we care about them and have compassion for them. The more we do this, the more we enhance rapport. Some of the everyday ways we can do this are to:

- run to time (or not far off) in clinic
- be consistent and reliable in all our dealings with young people and their families
- remember what we have been told in previous sessions
- follow up on things we said we would follow up on (e.g., sending them a link to a helpful app or podcast)
- ask about events in a child's life they told us were coming up (e.g., a birthday, going to a first gig, a holiday)
- apologize when we do or say something we know did not feel right for the young person.

Overall, even though we are professionals and should act as such, we also need to be human. I sometimes feel there is so much emphasis on "professionalism" that practitioners feel it is wrong to also show they are human beings. Of course, professional boundaries are of the upmost importance, but so too are spontaneous and heartfelt interactions. If you have not seen your six-year-old patient for a few weeks over the summer holidays, show that you are really excited to see him again. When your 13-year-old patient tells you they did really well in an exam they had been worried about, show them you are absolutely thrilled for them. When a young person you work with is having a difficult time, open your heart to them and sit with them in their pain as you would with a friend or a relative. This concept very much relates back to the idea of authenticity that I discussed in Chapter 1.

Seven steps to gaining and maintaining rapport

1. Being present
2. Starting with the person not the symptoms
3. Advance and retreat
4. Meeting the needs of the situation
5. Active listening
6. Understanding that every child needs something different
7. Care and compassion

Creating rapport with babies and toddlers

Most of the seven steps outlined above also apply to babies and toddlers, although in practice, how we enact them may look somewhat different. There is an added component to developing rapport with our youngest patients, however.

When you observe, for example, a contented eight-month-old baby, you will see that their *qi* is fluid and changeable and that they seem to respond almost entirely to the present moment. It's as if their *qi* is doing a little dance and has its own tune. The trick is for the practitioner to join the dance and be in sync with them. Musicians require a similar skill if they come on stage when the band is already playing and need to join in. A good musician will quickly find the rhythm and key the band are playing in and seamlessly join in with it. This is what we need to do with babies and toddlers—find their rhythm and get in sync and in tune with them. I find that as long as I am in sync, the little person will usually feel good about being with me and allow me to do my treatment.

Of the seven steps described above, the three that are most important when working with babies and toddlers are:

- Being present
- Advance and retreat
- Meeting the needs of the situation.

Creating rapport with teenagers

As well as the seven steps described above, there is one more point to make about creating and maintaining rapport with teenagers. Teens really need to feel that you are on their side. Many teens spend a lot of time feeling that either the world is against them or everybody is nagging them, or both. Many also develop a rather prickly exterior which means that it can be difficult for their loved ones to know how to convey their love to them in a way which is accepted.

It is perhaps easier to start by mentioning things we should avoid doing when working with teenagers. Here are some key "no-nos" when working with teens:

- Do not nag.
- Do not bombard them with lifestyle advice.
- Do not tell them their feelings are exaggerated.

- Do not grill them or force them to talk about their feelings if they are not ready to.
- Do not make assumptions about how they are feeling or why they are behaving in the ways they are.
- Do not necessarily collude with the messages that their parents want them to hear.

I find that one of the best ways to be with teens is simply to be quietly curious. If you follow the seven steps, they will sense that you care, that they can be themselves with you and that you want to work *with* them. Teens need to know you are on their team.

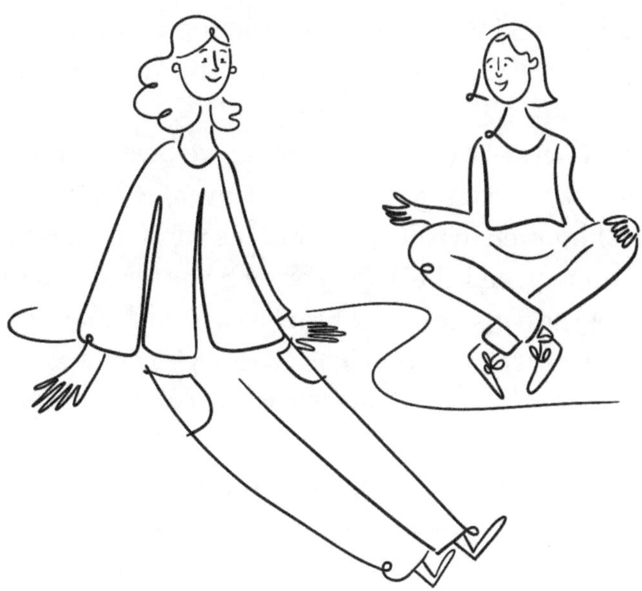

Troubleshooting

Problem: Two-year-old Grace arrives in my clinic extremely grumpy, having just woken up from a nap. Even my best efforts will not get her out of her grump. She simply needs time, but I have a full schedule and only 20 minutes of the appointment left.

Solution: This is where the concept of *wu wei* comes into its own. I may have had a wonderful plan of exactly what I wanted to do in that session, but sometimes the best course of action is to let go of the best laid plans. I ask myself, considering in this moment that little Grace does not want me anywhere near her, "How can I best use the time?" It may be that I can do the *tui na* I wanted to do on Grace on her mum, and her mum can simultaneously do it on Grace. Or it may be that I can mark some points on Grace and give her mum seeds or magnets to put on them when they get home. Or maybe this is a chance for Mum to talk through some worries she has, and I can listen and (if appropriate) make some suggestions. And, magically, it may be that once Grace no longer senses pressure to get out of her grump, she will in fact come round to allowing me to do some treatment on her. The key is to be flexible and gauge what the moment calls for.

Problem: Twelve-year-old Alice, who I've been treating for a while, is on the autism spectrum and arrives feeling furious. Her mum had forgotten to let her know in the morning that they had an appointment, and she is someone who needs to know things in advance. She curls up on the beanbag and continues to tell her mum how cross she is with her. Even though I know she usually enjoys her treatments, she says she doesn't want to be here and just wants to go home.

Solution: It is obvious to me that Alice's Liver *qi* has become jammed up in response to her day not being as she thought it would. If I become another person trying to get her to do something she doesn't want to, I suspect she will dig her heels in further. In contrast, if I give her some leeway, I hope her *qi* might relax a little. When Alice was younger, she used to enjoy having her treatments on the beanbag, although nowadays I always ask her to get on the treatment table. Today, as a one-off treat, I say she can have her treatment on the beanbag. This is not ideal from my point of view, but it allows Alice to feel she has some control or say in what is going to happen.

Problem: Fifteen-year-old Jacob arrives for his first session. He obviously has conflicting feelings about being here at all. His mum tells me that he sleeps really badly, and that is why they have come for treatment. He just sits there making "fed up" eyes at his mum and not wanting to engage with me at all.

Solution: At times like these, the best policy is often to name the awkwardness. I turn to Jacob and say, "I can see that you are unsure about being here. I really appreciate you turning up. First of all, it would be great to get to know you a little, and then for you to tell me in your own words about your sleep or anything else that is going on for you. I will let you know if and how I think I might be able to help. If you are willing to give me three or four sessions before making a decision about whether acupuncture is for you, that would be great." The key here is for me to connect with Jacob and let him know he has choices. I want him to know that it is not enough for me that his mum wants him to be here; I have to know that he does too.

Problem: Ten-year-old Ethan comes to me for treatment because of his school-related anxiety. He has not attended school since the Covid-19 pandemic, which was four years ago. He seems happy to let his mum do the talking, and when I ask him a question, he looks to her to answer it. He sits with his arms crossed and his legs curled up as if to protect himself. I am struggling to make a connection with him.

Solution: The concept of "advance and retreat" comes to mind with Ethan. If I advance too much or too quickly, he will curl up to protect himself even more. The key with Ethan is to go slowly. At the same time, I need to be mindful that I don't collude with the current pattern of him automatically looking to his mum to answer everything. So I try to balance his need for a slow move towards further connection with gentle encouragement for him to find his voice. I stay alert to key, opportune moments when I can draw him into the conversation.

Summary

Creating and maintaining rapport with all the young people who come to our clinics is probably one of the most challenging and yet also the most rewarding parts of being a pediatric acupuncturist. As we have discussed in this chapter, rapport enables us to treat a child and also turbocharges the efficacy of whichever treatment modalities we use.

There are also broader and more far-reaching benefits of the relationships we build with the little people we treat. As practitioners who may see them on and off throughout their childhood and adolescence, we are in the privileged position of being a trusted adult. We may know them, perhaps in a different way, but just as deeply as a family member. As we have some emotional distance, we may be the person they turn to as they come into their teenage years when turning to a close family member feels difficult.

As Francis Peabody said, "The secret of the care of the patient is in caring for the patient."[27]

CHAPTER 3

The Art of Creating a Relationship with Parents

Building a relationship with the parents of the children we treat comes second only to building a relationship with the child. Parents will not entrust the care of their child to you unless they feel confident in you as a practitioner. Of course, the parent (unless they themselves are an acupuncturist), will not actually *know* whether or not you are skilled at acupuncture. However, they need to *feel* that you know what you are doing. Your relationship with them will be shaped to a large degree by how well you communicate.

This begs the question of what you need to convey to a parent that constitutes "good communication." Reflecting on my own practice, I believe the key things a parent needs to feel are that:

- they trust you
- they have confidence in your skills and abilities as an acupuncturist
- you care enough to do your absolute best for their child
- you have empathy and compassion
- you are honest (especially in terms of expectations of treatment) and have integrity
- you are reliable and professional.

Before the appointment

How you communicate when a parent makes initial contact with you is often the deciding factor in terms of whether or not they will bring their child to you for treatment. This initial contact could be via email, a face-to-face video call or a standard phone call.

I offer parents a free 15-minute call before the child's initial appointment. During the call, I invite the parent to tell their child's story. The active listening described in Chapter 2 is important here as well. The parent needs to feel that I am listening mindfully and attentively to what they have to say. If I feel I can help, I will convey this, along with the degree to which I think I can help. I will also tell them very approximately how long I think it will take. This phone call is also an opportunity to ask the parent if there is anything I should know that they do not feel comfortable communicating in front of their child. This is important. We want to make sure that the child is not witness to their parent's anxiety. There may also be difficulties, either past or present, in the life of the family that they feel it is important to share but which may be inappropriate for the child to hear. If there is too much to say in a phone call, I invite the parent to email me before their child's first appointment. If I feel I can't help, I try my best to suggest somebody else who may be better suited to helping them, rather than leaving them feeling that they have reached the end of the line.

Parents find this initial call invaluable. Many of the parents who seek our help are desperate and feel that they do not have anywhere else to turn. Whilst we must avoid at all costs giving false hope, to offer a realistic sense of hope to the parent is in itself a gift.

A parent of a three-year-old rang me to see if I could help her son who suffered repeated respiratory infections. He often ended up being hospitalized, as he became severely breathless. I told her I thought I could help. Further down the line, she said that I was the first person who had ever said to her they thought they could help her son. Prior to this, doctors had just said they would have to wait until her son grew out of the problem. On hearing that there might be help and that this was not something they just needed to put up with, she said she took "a really deep breath" for the first time in years. I thought this was interesting. Knowing how much small children mirror their parents, maybe this phone call was actually the first stage in her son's healing journey. He responded well to treatment and, even when he did get an infection, never had to be hospitalized again.

I find there are certain sentiments that I express frequently during my initial phone calls with parents, for example:

- It sounds as if this has been very challenging for you all.
- I'm so sorry to hear your child is struggling in this way.
- I have helped many children with this kind of issue before, so I feel cautiously confident I will be able to help your child too.
- I have not seen this exact issue before but Chinese medicine is well suited to treating this kind of problem.
- Please reassure your child that I will go at their pace.
- Please reassure your child that there is no pressure to have needles, as I have many effective non-needle alternatives.

There are also certain questions that I frequently ask parents during these initial phone calls, such as:

- Is your child generally happy talking about this issue?
- Have you discussed with your child the possibility of

bringing them to see me? (With older children and teenagers, this is especially important.)
- Is there anything we haven't already spoken about that I should be aware of concerning how I interact with your child?
- Do you have any other questions or concerns?

Whatever format you choose to use, I highly recommend providing an option for parents to have 15 minutes or so of your time before you first see their child. This helps them but it also helps you. Having a sense beforehand of who you are going to be seeing and what type of issue they are struggling with enables you to prepare mentally and emotionally. It means you can begin your therapeutic relationship with the child and their parent on the right foot and that there are fewer "unknowns" during the initial session.

During the appointment

Assuming that I have already had some contact with the parent prior to the appointment, when I first meet the parent and child in the clinic, my priority is to make the child feel as comfortable as possible. However, the parent must feel welcome too, as must siblings and any other family members who come along for the ride. Parents may feel nervous. They may have concerns about whether they are doing the right thing for their child or about how their child will respond to being in your clinic. A warm and confident welcome from us will help to put them at ease.

I always have the parent in the room for the entire duration of the initial appointment (with the exception of older teenagers who express a preference for coming in without their parent*). Most children feel much more comfortable having a parent in

* Practitioners must be sure to follow the guidelines of their professional body in terms of at what age they are able to have the child in the room on their own.

the room with them. However, there are other reasons for having the parent there too. On a practical level, the parent will be able to give us information about the child's early life, the pregnancy and birth, etc. On an emotional level, it sets the tone that the three of us (or four of us if both parents are there) are going to work together as a team.

The real skill during appointments is to be able to create rapport with both the child and the parent. We need to give them both a space to voice what needs to be said and actively listen to them both. We need to manage the balance of who is taking up the space. Of course, how we do this is hugely dependent on the age of the child, as well as the personalities of both the parent and child. We must be constantly vigilant as to how both the parent and child are feeling. Is the child feeling sidelined? Is the parent feeling ignored? A well-known phrase often attributed to John Lydgate tells us, "You can please some of the people all of the time, you can please all of the people some of the time but you can't please all of the people all of the time." As pediatric acupuncturists, however, that is exactly what we have to try to do.

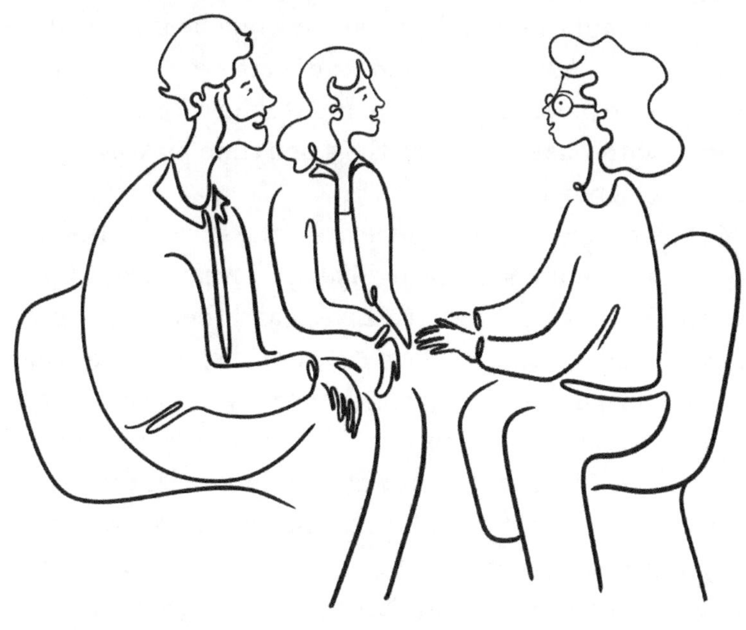

Some guiding principles

When navigating our way through the complexities of managing dynamics and relationships within the treatment room, I use the following guiding principles as my compass:

- The child is our patient, and our primary responsibility is to do what is best for them.
- The parent loves their child and should always be heard, taken into account and treated with compassion.
- I am the professional and ultimately need to act in a way which is aligned with my professional and moral judgment.

The best way to illustrate how you might go about navigating the relationship with the parent in the child's treatment is to give some examples from my own practice.

Five-year-old Luke and his mum

Luke is a very confident and articulate five-year-old who suffers from asthma. Mum is very talkative and somewhat anxious. Luke really enjoys his appointments but at times gets frustrated because his mum keeps talking to me while he is trying to tell me something and whilst he and I are "in the zone" together. My challenge is to prevent Mum from interfering with my treatment dynamic with Luke, whilst at the same time making sure she doesn't feel ignored.

My solution is to be super clear! At the start of the session, I say to Luke's mum something like, "I'd love to hear from you how you feel Luke has been this week and then after (turning to Luke) I want to hear from you." Before I begin the treatment, I say to Luke's mum, "I'm going to turn my attention solely to Luke now but if there is anything else that feels important for you to tell me, I'd love to hear it when I've finished the treatment." If Luke's mum does start talking to me during the treatment, I gently and warmly remind her that I will come to her when I've finished. Sometimes, I simply don't respond to her but when this happens, I always make sure to check in with her afterwards and say, "I think there was something else that you wanted to say."

Fourteen-year-old May and her mum

May and her mum come in for the initial session. May suffers from intense period pains. She and her mum are in a difficult place in their relationship. Every time Mum opens her mouth, May rolls her eyes, tells her she is wrong, huffs and puffs and says something like, "What's the point, you just don't understand me at all." My challenge is to make a connection with May without colluding with her rejection of her mum.

As May is 14, I trust that she can give me most of the key information I need herself. So I suggest to her and her mum that rather than having a three-way conversation, I direct my questions solely at May first, and she can answer them on her own. I then suggest to May that, while I understand she and her mum have different views, her mum's perspective is also valuable, so afterwards, we allow her mum to have her say. I reassure May that my priority is her and helping her to feel better.

Seven-year-old Tristan and his dad

Tristan is coming to see me because he is having problems with emotional regulation. He likes his dad to be near him while he has his treatment so that he can hold his hand. Dad sits beside him and likes to answer his emails and make some business calls during the session. As Tristan feels his dad's attention go elsewhere, he plays up more and more, and it makes it hard to carry out the treatment. My challenge is to communicate to Dad that Tristan would really benefit from having his undivided attention during the session. Dad is clearly a "type A" personality who I suspect will find it a challenge to simply be there for Tristan and switch off from business.

I decide to speak directly and honestly with Dad, imagining that he is used to direct communication in his working life. Before we start treatment, I tell him that we need to do things differently to last time. I explain that I feel Tristan gets confused when his dad is physically there but preoccupied with work and that it means I can't give him the treatment he needs. I suggest that what works really well with many children is for their parent to read to them while they have their treatment, and I hand him a book I think Tristan will like. I have calculated that he won't physically be able to both hold a book up for Tristan and do stuff on his phone, so this is a better option than simply suggesting he talks to Tristan. This is a win-win situation. Tristan gets what he needs from his dad, I can carry out treatment and Dad gets to see how happy Tristan is when he gives him his undivided attention.

Between appointments

My belief is that part of my role in looking after children involves communicating with parents between appointments. Parents will have queries or concerns, their child's condition will change or they might want clarification on something we mentioned during treatment. However, I also believe that it's important I set clear boundaries as to how and when I am happy to be contacted. I want to be available but am by no means "open all hours."

It is for each individual practitioner to decide what their limits are and what they feel happy with. Everybody's circumstances will differ. My aim is to be flexible but not to my own detriment. I aim to have clear boundaries but not to the extent that parents feel that I am inaccessible.

My general rule of thumb is that I am happy to have brief email or message contact between appointments whenever necessary. I let parents know that I will respond to them as soon as I can, although that might not always be immediately. I consider this extra "out of hours" time to be a part of what they pay me for and included in my treatment fee. However, if we need to have longer, more in-depth discussions about their child, I ask them to book in an online session with me via my website for which I will charge.

It is, of course, necessary to make it clear to parents from the outset that if they have an immediate, serious concern about their child's health, they should contact a medical healthcare professional.

Communication between appointments is often initiated by the parent but may also be initiated by me. This is especially the case if I am working with an older child or teenager who comes into the treatment room on their own. I may want to get the parent's perspective on how their child is doing, knowing that I may not be getting the whole picture from the child themselves. Or I may want to touch base with a parent and keep them up to date with my perspective of how treatment is going. Of course, it is always necessary to communicate with a parent without breaking the confidence of the child or teen, except in cases where we are concerned for the young person's safety or the safety of others.

In my experience, parents really appreciate this "in between" communication. It helps them to feel supported in the face of their child's struggles. It also reminds them that I care for and am doing the best I can for their child.

Troubleshooting

Let's have a look at some commonly occurring situations that need particular thought.

The anxious parent

Illness in a child, both physical, mental and emotional, is extremely hard for parents. It can trigger a huge range of emotions, one of which is anxiety. As the child's practitioner, the parent often sees us as someone to whom they can offload their anxiety. How we respond to this is important, both for them and for us.

For the parent, never underestimate the power of listening. Simply listening well is often all we need to do. Although we may be able to make some helpful suggestions, these can wait until after we have listened. Many parents tell me that I am the first person who has taken their concerns seriously and not dismissed them as "just being an anxious parent." This in itself is powerful.

For the practitioner, being on the receiving end of the parent's anxiety can have its challenges. We should try to avoid feeling responsible at one end of the spectrum, and dismissive and uncaring at the other end. The middle ground is to feel compassion. Whilst we want to help, that does not mean it's our job to fix everything. Whilst we care, we must remain separate to and outside of the problem.

Crucially, when managing an anxious parent, we must make sure that we try as far as possible to keep their anxiety outside of the treatment room. It should not be expressed in front of the child any more than is absolutely necessary. This may involve gently yet firmly stopping the parent mid-sentence and saying something like, "I understand this is really difficult for you. I'd like to find a different time to hear your concerns so that I can fully focus on your child now." I may then ask a parent to book an online session with me where I can give them time to voice their feelings, listen to them, suggest a way forward and also make it clear to them that it's best for their child to keep these feelings out of the treatment room.

There are occasions when it feels appropriate to signpost parents to other sources of support, such as a counsellor or a therapist. Just as we need to always be mindful of when to bring in wider support for the child, the same goes for the parent.

The "other" parent

We have so far discussed dealing with one parent. The reality is that it is most commonly one parent who brings their child for an appointment. Whether the parents are together or not, there is usually a second parent.

When we first meet the "other" parent, they are often curious and excited to see their child having their acupuncture appointment, about which they may have heard a lot. However, sometimes they may be skeptical or less inclined towards acupuncture than the parent we usually see. That's OK. If I sense a certain dismissiveness or disbelief, rather than trying to show them or even prove to them that what I am doing is of value, I just focus, as always, on giving the child the best treatment I can. Let the medicine talk for you. I have had many a skeptical parent leave an appointment better disposed towards acupuncture than when they came. Even when this doesn't happen, if they feel good about *you* and the way you interact with and care for their child, then it is a win.

Nine-year-old Arthur was usually brought for treatment to my multibed clinic by his mum, but several months into treatment his dad brought him. Arthur was a shy and quiet boy, but the team and I had developed a really strong bond with him, and he always chatted away to us happily throughout his treatment. At the end of his session, Arthur's dad told me that he didn't know whether acupuncture "worked" or not but that it warmed his heart to see his son come out of his shell and communicate with us in the way he did. Rather than feeling offended by his ambivalence towards acupuncture, I felt happy that he had seen a side of his son during the appointment that he hadn't previously known was possible.

You feel that the parent is a part of the problem

Parents are usually doing their very best for their children 99.9% of the time, sometimes in extremely difficult circumstances. However, we all bring to parenting the hurts and wounds from our own childhoods, as well as our particular emotional proclivities. Our past informs how we respond to our children and sometimes means we respond in a way that is not helpful for them. There is no blame or judgment here. However, there are times as a practitioner when we feel that the parent's behavior or dynamic with their child is exacerbating the child's struggles or preventing them from getting better.

Let's take a specific example from my clinic. Aimee is the mother of three-year-old Dylan, a sensitive boy who becomes more and more hyperactive and tricky to manage the more he senses his mother's anxiety. During Dylan's sessions, I saw clearly that the more anxious Aimee became about Dylan's "acting up," the more Dylan would act up. Aimee would often say things in front of Dylan such as, "What have I done wrong that he starts playing up like this?" or, "I just can't handle this kind of behavior," always spoken in a hugely anxious tone. Children need to feel that their parents can manage their behavior and emotions. When we respond to them in an intensely emotional way, especially at Dylan's tender age, it makes them feel unsafe.

When I notice this kind of unhelpful dynamic, my approach is to foster two qualities towards the parent: empathy and curiosity. The first, empathy, is needed because finding yourself in a situation where the particular struggles of your child trigger a deep and intense emotion in you is painful and sometimes excruciating. The second, curiosity, is needed because when we understand something, we can more easily forgive it on the one hand and support the parent with it on the other hand.

I asked Aimee if she would be happy to have a session with me without Dylan. During the session, Aimee shared with me aspects of her difficult childhood and her feelings that she was failing as a mother. Whenever Dylan got upset or cross or struggled to manage his emotions, Aimee was hit with a deep sense that she had failed. This caused her huge amounts of anxiety, which Dylan sensed and which then exacerbated his behavior.

Together, Aimee and I made a plan. First, I signposted her to a local parent support group. Second, we agreed that during Dylan's sessions, Aimee would sit and read a book or magazine and let me interact with Dylan on my own. This gave her a chance to untangle herself from their tricky dynamic temporarily and to have "time out" from feeling responsible. Third, I taught Aimee some breathing exercises to do whenever she felt her anxiety rising during a difficult interaction with Dylan.

As acupuncturists, we are not taught how to deal with these types of situations. They are not easy at all. Yet we must *always* be guided by what is best for the child, so it is beholden on us to address anything that we see is strongly and negatively impacting them.

The parent feels their child needs treatment; you disagree

Over the years, I have been asked several times to treat a child who I believe does not need treatment. To some degree, of course, there is probably always something useful we can do to help a child, even one who is relatively well. However, when I get the sense that the parent wants their child to be treated because there is something about the child they want changed, I will not collude. Sometimes, there is a fine line between personality and pathology, but I will not treat a child simply because their parent wants them to be "different." This becomes even more the case if the child really does not enjoy the treatment (a likely scenario if they feel they are being brought to you because their parent wants them to be someone they are not). What I may do in this case is to gently educate the parent on the nature of their child, explaining it through a Five Phase lens.

Treatment is not going well

If a child is not responding to treatment in the way that you, they or their parent hoped, the best thing to do is to talk about it. Try to avoid it becoming the elephant in the room. You might say something like, "I am aware that we have not yet got the results we were all hoping for." In my experience, this kind of honesty is usually appreciated. Find out how the parents and child are feeling about treatment. Delve deeper and ask more questions. If you have any, let them know your thoughts about why you are not having more success. Together, make a plan of action. Finally, communicate to the family when you feel that there is no point in continuing treatment. How we act and communicate when we have not been able to help someone is as important, if not more so, than when things are going well.

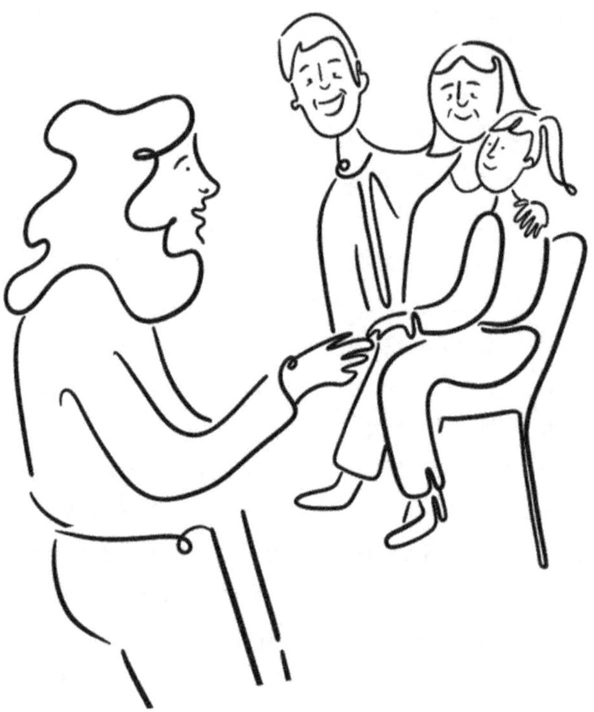

Summary

Communicating with parents is a central part of working with children. In order to help the child, we need to cultivate a good relationship with one or both parents. I endeavor to create a team spirit. The three (or four) of us are all working together with one aim in mind—to help the child. Communicating well with parents, at times reassuring them, sometimes offering helpful suggestions, when necessary talking with them on their own, may all be part of what helps a child to heal, alongside the treatment we give to the child directly. A parent and young child, are a "*qi* bubble."* They are one unit and therefore we need to support the unit as a whole. I would also argue that even a parent and a teenage child are still energetically inextricably linked. Each is affected by what happens to the other. Parents need our kindness, our compassion and our consideration. Honing our skills in communicating with them is an essential part of what we do.

* I first heard this wonderful phrase from my colleague and friend Elisa Rossi.

CHAPTER 4

The Art of Working with Families and Their Dynamics

Everyone who comes for acupuncture, whether adult or child, is part of a family, whether that be a birth family, the family they grew up with and/or the one they have created as an adult. However, one of the things that sets pediatrics apart is the fact that the children we see are actively connected to their family. As they grow, they are being shaped by the dynamics of the family, as well as by the wider society of which they are a part. This is inherently neither "good" nor "bad'; it is simply an unavoidable truth. The better appreciation and understanding we have of this, the more we can help the child. In the *Lü Shi Chun Qiu* of 239 BC we read:

> All phenomena have their causes. If one does not know these causes, although one may happen to be right about the facts, it is as if one knew nothing and in the end one will be bewildered.[28]

If a child comes to us with recurrent headaches, we can understand their headaches in terms of TEAMs pathology. Perhaps their Liver blood is weak and not rooting Liver *yang*, for example. This may be accurate, but it is also limited. The fact that their headaches began when their dad lost his job or that they come more frequently when Mum is away are equally important pieces of the jigsaw. When we are able to put together the whole picture, we will treat a child more confidently, more holistically and ultimately more successfully.

The aim of this chapter is to create awareness of the family dynamics and their impact on children. At the end, I suggest strategies for how to manage this in your work.

The importance of family relationships

Wang Fengyi (1864–1937) was a Confucian educator from northern China. He developed a deep understanding of how emotional patterns rooted in family relationships can manifest in chronic disease. His follower, Liu Yousheng wrote:

> Don't talk of mysteries! Don't talk of subtlety! Focus your teaching on the Dao of being human. And where does this Dao of being human start? It starts with the five relationships. It starts with the family. Family relationships are the crucial step in the Dao![29]

Family relationships are a large part of what forms us. When we treat children, we do not treat them in isolation but we treat them as part of a family unit. What is going on in this family unit can impact when and how a child gets ill and how their illness manifests, as well as over what period of time they may recover.

Family dynamics get played out in our treatment room

It's not uncommon to hear parents in the treatment room say things such as, "Where has this behavior come from?" There seems to be something about being in a contained space, with a non-family adult there, that allows emotions to come to the surface or dynamics to be played out. Some children sense that it is a safe place to allow things out that they keep hidden away at home. This may be the expression of a difficult emotion towards the parent or of siblings having a big spat. Or it could be an outpouring of tears or suddenly letting out a secret that the parent had no idea about.

When this happens, a parent's first response is often to apologize on behalf of their child. While there are times when we have to draw firm boundaries around behavior, I always welcome the expression of emotion in my clinic. I reassure parents that it is not a problem at all for their child to be expressing powerful emotions. I often also mention to them that it's common for this to happen in this setting.

Mostly, however, when these dynamics come to the surface, our job is to hold the space and keenly observe. Emotions are information. In TEAMs, they are known as the internal causes of disease, and when they are intense, prolonged or repressed, they negatively impact the balance of *qi* in the body. Moreover, they help us to understand more deeply how we can best support the child not only with our treatment but also with our presence.

Whilst we are not family therapists, we can play a role in supporting a shift in an unhelpful dynamic. Here are a few examples of how we might do this:

- Provide a safe space to allow anything that needs to be expressed.
- Encourage both the parent and child to listen to each other.
- Endeavor to hold a non-partisan position in which we mediate between the parent and child, or between siblings, without judgment or favor.

These moments when family dynamics and intense emotions come to the surface are all moments of opportunity. Expression is a way of moving stuck *qi*. It causes knots to come undone and allows for change and progress. If we can remain unruffled and centered amidst this intensity, we are doing the young person a great service.

Family dynamics and chronic illness

When little people are struggling with their health, the ramifications are enormous. The child themselves may become more needy, sensitive or angry. Their friendships may suffer as they have time off school or can no longer attend clubs. Their physical and emotional development may be impacted when the illness lasts for some time.

Each parent may respond differently to the child's illness, which means their relationship may come under strain. Mum thinks the child should take the medications the doctor suggested; Dad is concerned about the possible side effects and wants to hold off. Someone needs to stay at home and look after the child who cannot go to school. Siblings may feel that the poorly child is taking the lion's share of their parents' time and attention. The emotional intensity in the household may go up a notch, which then negatively impacts the health of the child who is struggling. In short, when a child comes to our clinic, they are often at the center of a messy, complex and confusing web of emotional patterns and family intricacies. We cannot untangle all these knots, but having an awareness of them helps us to understand the child's predicament more fully.

The emotional milieu of the family

Do you remember as a child enjoying and feeling comfortable in the houses of some of your friends and in others never quite being able to relax? You may not have been able to explain it at the time, but this was most likely because you were picking up on the differing emotional environments. Children are like emotional sponges. It's as if they come into the world with a pair of strong antennae, which pick up on the nature of the *qi* which surrounds them. Some children, especially the more *xu*, deficient type children, do this more than others. However, all children pick up on and are molded and shaped by the environment in which they grow up.

Dr. Gabor Maté explains this perfectly when he says:

> Of all environments, the one that most profoundly shapes the human personality is the invisible one: the emotional atmosphere in which the child lives during the critical early years. The invisible environment has little to do with parenting philosophies or parenting style. It is a matter of intangibles, foremost among them being the parents' relationship with each other and their emotional balance as individuals.[30]

Emotions are *qi*. Families and households have their own unique "flavor" of *qi*. If there is a lot of worry, sadness, hidden anger, overt conflict or agitation, to name but a few possibilities, the *qi* of the household will become colored by that. Just as stuck or intense emotions in the body affect the movements of *qi* in the *zangfu*, so too do they affect the *qi* of the external environment. This has a profound effect on the *qi* of the children living in that environment. On the positive side, good *qi* environments can protect children against illness and help them to heal if they do succumb. On the negative side, bad *qi* environments can trigger or perpetuate illness.

The Five Phase family

All the members of a household are interlinked and impact on each other in ways which may sometimes be obvious but often happen without anybody really realizing it.

Let's take a look at what this means in daily life. We will use the Shen family as our model. The Shen family contains Mum (Joan), Dad (John), 14-year-old Jed, eight-year-old Josie and three-year-old Jane.

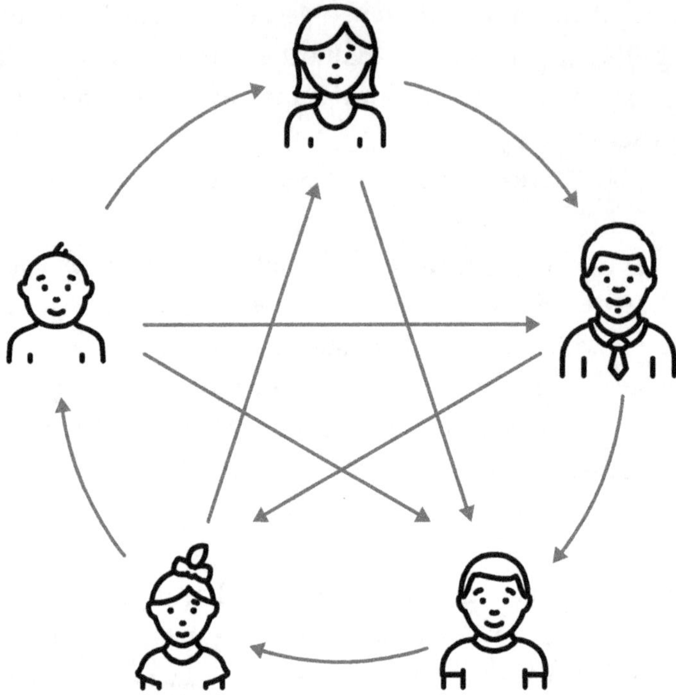

DIAGRAM 4.1 THE FIVE PHASES AND THE FAMILY

Mum Joan is a Fire type. She is naturally bubbly and affectionate with her children. Joan is very easily hurt, however, and feels rather unloved in her relationship with John. John is a Metal type and, while he loves Joan dearly, he finds it hard to express this to her, and Joan spends a lot of time feeling upset. It doesn't help that 14-year-old Jed is a Wood type, as well as being in the midst of adolescent changes. Jed doesn't have as much freedom as he would like, and most days there is at least one time when he screams and shouts at his parents and runs out of the room slamming the door behind him. Joan feels very hurt by this and would love John to comfort her. John, as is the way with a lot of Metal types, perceives it as a personal failure that his son acts in this way and responds by withdrawing and hiding in his home office behind his work.

Josie is a Water type. She has been suffering from recurrent bladder infections since she was five years old. Josie has always been the one in the family to be most affected by the emotional environment. She feels anxious and agitated when Jed shouts or when she senses that her mum is feeling sad. Her parents have always noticed that Josie can only truly relax when everyone in the family is happy and harmonious. Her bladder infections have become more frequent since Jed became a teenager and the tension in the family increased.

The baby of the family, Jane, was born six weeks prematurely. She had some health complications as a result and was in and out of hospital for the first year of her life. This was obviously a stressful time for everyone, but Josie (who was five at the time) found it especially hard. If she had been able to express it at such a young age, she would have said that she felt insecure, as if her security blanket had been taken away from her. She was used to Mum and Dad mainly being at home and emotionally available to her, and after Jane's birth, they were often either physically absent or emotionally absent, or both. Her response, as a Water child, was to feel fearful.

Reading about the Shen family, we may ask ourselves the question—are Josie's bladder infections *caused by* the difficult time after the birth of her little sister, her brother being a moody teenager and her mum and dad not feeling connected? Strictly speaking, the answer to this is probably no. But what we *can* say is that these family dynamics are in the mix and contribute to the problem. Josie's constitution has caused her to interact and respond to the events of her life in a particular way, which has predisposed her to bladder infections. We can also say that the bladder infections are, in one sense, a way that Josie is expressing her feelings of fear and insecurity. What happens to one family member will impact the whole family.

Qi knots

Even when they are mainly healthy, family relationships often have knotty aspects to them. I like to call these "*qi* knots." *Qi* knots tend to arise when certain emotions cannot be expressed, for whatever reason. They may also arise when family members get stuck in an emotion. They may appear when a parent and child seem to trigger intense feelings in the other, often in one particular area of life. A certain amount of "knottiness" is part and parcel of family life, but when these knots become really tight, they can contribute to illnesses becoming chronic and can prevent a child from getting better.

Ten-year-old Loretta wet the bed every night but also had accidents during the day. Her mum felt that these daytime accidents were mainly because Loretta got distracted by what she was doing and didn't recognize that she needed to urinate. So when they were at home, Mum would suggest to Loretta every 30 minutes or so that she go to the toilet to see if she needed a wee. Whilst this was a perfectly reasonable thing for Loretta's mum to do, Loretta said it made her feel as if her mum was treating her like a toddler and it really angered her. Loretta's mum, in response, felt angry because it often meant she had to deal with the fall out of Loretta having an accident. The two were locked in anger around this issue. It seemed to me that Loretta, in part, continued to wet herself during the day to get at her mum. Having an accident became a way of communicating her anger with her mum. The two were locked in a *qi* knot which had become a part of what perpetuated Loretta's condition. This did not directly change my treatment of Loretta but it influenced how I communicated with her. For example, we agreed she would set a timer on one of her devices every 30 minutes, which would remind her to go to the toilet, instead of her mum having to remind her. This helped to separate her urinary issue from her relationship with her mum.

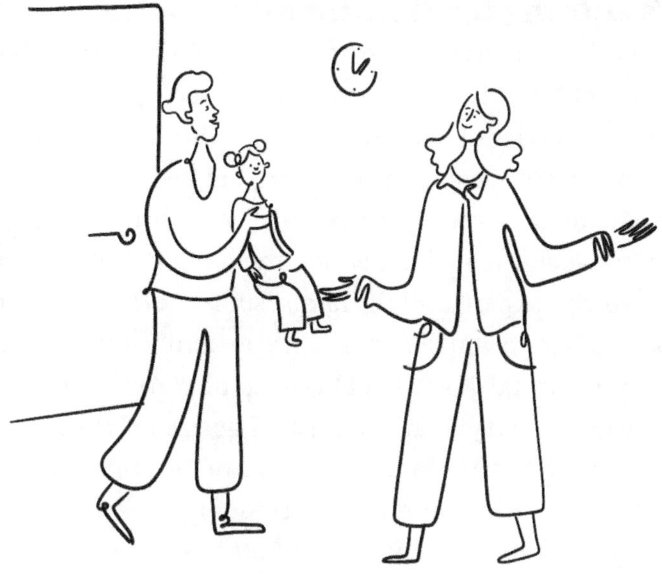

The family scapegoat

Sometimes, the child who is being brought for treatment is the family scapegoat. They are blamed in some way for the problems of the family. For example, recently a parent said to me of their child, "Johnnie just makes things difficult for all of us with his anger and defiance. His brother on the other hand does not have a bad bone in his body." Whilst it may well be that Johnnie has a naturally more Woody temperament than his brother, it is also likely that he is being unfairly blamed for the problems in the family. It can be easier to scapegoat than to look at the family system. Johnnie may be sensing that he is less loved and more easily criticized or blamed than his brother, which would only increase his tendency to anger and defiance. It could also be that Johnnie's mother is particularly intolerant of expressions of anger, perhaps related to her own family dynamics as a child. So she finds him less easy to love than his naturally softer brother.

Who's coming for treatment?

So, as a result of everything we have discussed so far in this chapter, when a child arrives in our treatment room, they bring with them the energetics of the whole family. There may be one child and one parent physically in the room, but the energetics of the household are there too. This may take the form of an unspoken tension between the parents which the child has absorbed, or a sadness which has pervaded the family since the death of a sibling, or a financial strain which hangs over the family like a cloud, suppressing the natural, joyous bubbling up of *qi*. We need to hold a sense of this as we try to understand what has led the child to be ill or perpetuated their illness. Of course, many families are "good enough," and not all childhood conditions are rooted in the family dynamic. However, when they are, it helps to be aware of it.

Five-year-old Melissa was lashing out at other children at school, throwing things around the classroom and biting. Her mother was distraught, as she didn't feel this was in keeping with Melissa's true nature. Melissa was always a lot calmer after her treatments, but four or five days later, the difficult behavior would return. I organized a Zoom session with Mum, as I instinctively felt there was something in Melissa's environment which was a part of the picture. Her Mum shared with me that her relationship with Melissa's father was at breaking point. They barely spoke to each other at home and, when they did, it usually ended up in an argument. Here was my answer. Melissa was absorbing the huge tension between her parents and then letting it out at school when she was in a different environment. I, of course, was not in a position to change the parental relationship, but knowing about it meant I could adapt my expectations of how Melissa would respond to her treatment and also explain this to her mum.

What do we do about family dynamics?

All of this begs the very important question of what we, as practitioners, do about these family dynamics. We may observe them, suspect them or intuit that they are there. Sometimes, as in the case of Melissa, we may be told about them overtly. Yet we are acupuncturists, not family therapists! So what do we do with this information?

- **Be observant**: The more we understand the context of the child's problems, the better we can support them. Having an awareness of the nuances and complexities of the situation helps to hone our intention and clarity in terms of treatment. The more insight we have into a situation, the more skilled we become at bringing about a change.

- **Keep your focus on the child**: There is usually little we can do to directly change the dynamics within a family, and that is not our job anyway. However, what we can do is help the child to be in the best place possible in order to withstand the dynamic. For example, going back to the Shen family, the more we support Josie's Kidneys and Water phase as a whole, the less insecure she will feel in the face of her brother's anger and her parents' difficulties. Crucially, the stronger her Kidney *qi*, the less susceptible she will become to bladder infections.

- **When possible, communicate with the parents**: It is amazing how powerful and transformative it can be to simply provide a space for a parent to talk about what is difficult within the family. Once again, we are not family therapists, so we do not need to respond in the way a therapist would. We simply need to actively listen and respond with compassion. Allowing a parent to get something off their chest can shift blocked *qi*. As the parent and child's *qi* is interlinked, this alone can bring about a shift in the child too.

- **Stay mindful of opportunities to gently present a different viewpoint**: Can you help a parent to see that their child may be expressing anger but feeling unloved underneath it? Or that the problem is not solely with them but that they are acting out a problem with the family system? Can you point out that because of their Five Phase constitution, they need something different to a sibling?

- **Modify your expectations**: The more we understand the context, the more accurate a prognosis we can make. To go back to our example of Melissa, I knew that until such time as her parents resolved their difficulties or separated, my treatments would only be able to help to a certain degree. Although over time I could help Melissa become more resilient to the less-than-ideal circumstances, it was not realistic to expect that she would not be continually harmed by them. It is akin to coming up against a strong external pathogenic factor. However good our *wei qi*, there are some pathogens that we will never be able to resist. Our job is to lessen the impact of the pathogen.

- **When necessary, signpost families to more support**: We cannot, and should not, be everything to everyone. There are certain situations and times when we may feel that the child, and the whole family, would benefit from having other medical healthcare professionals on board, such as a family therapist, a social worker or counsellor.

- **Watch out for magical things happening**: When we treat one child in the family, there may be ripple effects around the family. This is no different to treating the *zangfu* of the Wood phase, for example, and seeing an effect in the Earth phase. It is impossible to overstate the importance of focusing on the child and treating them to the best of our ability. Not always but sometimes, this triggers what can seem like a minor miracle.

Tommy, who suffered from bad tics, was always brought for treatments by his dad. Dad was a very successful guy professionally, and during Tommy's treatments, I noticed he also had big ambitions for Tommy. He would say things such as, "I just know you are going to be the top goal scorer in your game at the weekend," or, "You can definitely make it into that top math set." Whilst I am sure he only meant to be encouraging, I would see Tommy slump and look down in response to these comments, as if they just made him feel inadequate.

After a few sessions, I began to observe changes not only in Tommy but in his dad too. Whereas initially Dad would do a lot of talking and seemed to struggle to contain his exuberant energy during Tommy's sessions, he began to relax. During one particular treatment, Tommy lay very peacefully while having his treatment and Dad sat really quietly too, at times gently closing his eyes. Afterwards, he said it was a joy to see Tommy so relaxed and that that made him feel relaxed too. By the time Tommy had stopped coming for treatments, his dad had entirely refrained from his "motivational" comments towards Tommy. and they both seemed a lot easier in each other's company.

Tommy's case is an example of how treating one member of the family can impact another member, especially when they are the one in the treatment room with the child.

Summary

A friend of mine has a sign on the inside of their front door which reads, "Remember: as far as everyone else knows, we are a nice, normal family." This makes me laugh every time I see it. The only "normal" thing about any family is the wonderful complexity and messiness of it, hopefully alongside a whole lot of love too. Loving intensely and living alongside people we have been thrust together with is never going to be straightforward. When we work with children, we see this day in and day out. The tangles and knots that inevitably exist affect a child's health just as much as any other cause of disease, such as the climate, diet or the balance of work and rest. Whilst we can never eliminate all causes of disease, the more we are aware of them, the more effectively we can treat the child.

Finally, putting all these *qi* knots and tricky family dynamics to one side, what I am most struck by in my practice is the degree and power of love that exists between family members, even in the face of the most unbelievable stress and difficulty. Although the messiness may exacerbate or perpetuate a child's ill health, it is the love they receive that heals them.

Chapter 5

The Art of Working with Atypical Children

It is simplistic to suggest that there is such a thing as a "typical" child. Every child has a uniqueness that should be cherished and encouraged to be expressed. However, there are children for whom the approach described so far in this book will not be quite enough and who need an added layer of sensitivity and consideration. This chapter is a guide for practitioners working with these children.

Treating children with mental health difficulties

For a detailed approach to the treatment of child and teen anxiety and depression, please refer to Chapter 40 of *Acupuncture for Babies, Children and Teenagers* by Rebecca Avern.

Approximately 60% of all the children I see are primarily seeking treatment for varying degrees of mental health difficulties. This number has risen fast since the lockdowns resulting from the Covid-19 pandemic of 2020. These difficulties often manifest with anxiety, depression, self-harm or disordered eating. Some of these young people continue to function. They go to school, and they keep life together. Yet they are not thriving and are just managing and getting by. Others have stopped going to school, partaking in any social activities or even engaging in family life. It is tragic and awful that so many young people are struggling in this way. At the same time, it is wonderful that more and more are finding their way to acupuncture. There is so much we can do to help. Below I outline some general guidelines to take into account when treating young people with mental health difficulties.

Ensuring 360-degree support

Whilst I believe that acupuncture and related techniques are one of the most powerful ways to support young people struggling with their mental health, it may not always be enough on its own. For the sake of the young person, and for our sake, we may need to make sure there are other healthcare practitioners on board. This is especially important when we are working with young people who:

- have severely disordered eating
- have suicidal tendencies
- are struggling with addictions
- have a history of severe trauma.

Silence is golden

It's useful to remind yourself that, for some young people, just turning up to the appointment is a major achievement. I see teenagers who barely ever leave the house and for whom the idea of relating to someone they don't know fills them with anxiety. With this in mind, it is not always the right thing to do to try to get the young person to talk and open up to us. I feel that sometimes we fear we are not being a "good" practitioner if we don't achieve this. Yet, for some teens, this would be too much too soon, and if they feel pressure to talk, they will clam up and not come back. Keep in mind the idea of "advance and retreat" that is outlined in Chapter 2.

Of course, if the young person wants to talk, then that is fine and wonderful. If, however, they are not ready to do this, then we as acupuncturists are in the wonderful position of having other methods of diagnosis to call upon. Many young people who come to my clinic have already seen a counsellor or a therapist, but it hasn't suited them. We can use our skills of observation and palpation, for example, which will give us enough information to be able to form a diagnosis and carry out a treatment.

I treated a 14-year-old girl who did not say one word for the first two months of treatment. She would nod or shake her head, and in that way could give me consent to treat her. Then she began writing things down for me to read. She would hand me notes at the start of the sessions telling me how she felt. After a while, she started to say the odd word; for example, giving one-word answers to any questions. Over time, she communicated verbally more and more. I still see her today, and she is now one of the most expressive and articulate teenagers I know. Had I pushed her too much too soon, I suspect she would have stopped coming for treatment a long time ago.

Treat what you find

Sometimes, we might feel we need to do something different or extra when treating a young person with serious mental health problems. Perhaps this is because of a heightened sense of responsibility or because of a sense of urgency to "fix the problem." The phrase "more haste, less speed" comes to mind. Yet, as with anyone we are treating, we just need to focus on the patterns of imbalance we find and do our best to bring the child to a place of better balance.

How we go about treating the patterns of imbalance may be slightly different than if we were treating a purely physical issue. For example, we may use finer needles or choose more points which have a particular affinity with the *shen*. Apart from that, however, we just need to be even more aware of the importance of rapport and relationship (as discussed in Chapter 2).

Patience and presence

It can happen that a teen who is beset by worry or living with a chronically low mood, feels considerably better after only a small number of treatments. For example, when we strengthen the Spleen, the tendency to worry abates, or when we nourish the Heart, the mood may lift. However, with more complex mental health difficulties, treatment will take more time. When the *shen* has been impacted to the degree that the child is feeling the need to harm themselves or deny themselves food, there may be more to unpack, and that will take time.

One of the challenges of being a pediatric practitioner is learning to hold and stay present with the young person we are trying to help whilst they struggle. With complex mental health difficulties, that will take some time, and there may well be ups and downs along the way, especially in the midst of a tumultuous adolescence.

Managing our feelings of responsibility

One of the things that sets apart treating children from treating adults, is a child's inherent vulnerability. A child with mental health difficulties is even more vulnerable. Most of us go into this profession because we want to get people better, and this can at times make it difficult to stay present with the young person in the depths of their struggles. I find that what can make this more difficult is me feeling that I am responsible. If we feel we are responsible and a child is not doing well, it can create quite intense discomfort. Whilst we do have a responsibility—to care for and treat the young person to the best of our ability—this is not the same as being responsible overall. We can be a force for good in the child's life, but they will be subject to many other forces too, both good and bad. Our challenge is to remain present and patient whilst we do our bit to guide the young person towards health.

Liaising with parents

In Chapter 3, I discussed some aspects of communicating with parents. This subject deserves another mention in the context of mental health difficulties. Seeing your child struggle with their mental and emotional health is one of the most painful experiences a parent can have. As a result of this, I feel that we have some duty to look after the parent to some degree too, in the context of caring for their child.

If the parent does not stay in the room during the sessions, they may be concerned about how things are going in the treatment and keen to be kept in the loop. Whilst we cannot break their child's confidence (unless we are concerned about the safety of the child or others), we can offer them generalized updates. With the child's consent, I also like to ask parents for their observations of how their child is doing.

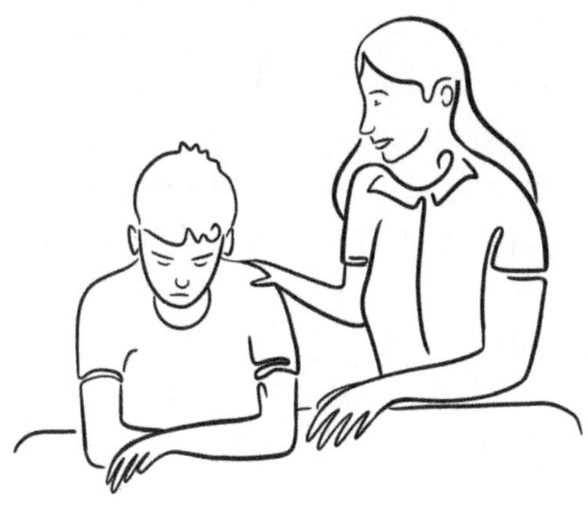

I frequently suggest to parents who I can see are struggling that they get some support themselves, and I have a range of acupuncturists and therapists I recommend. In TEAMs, we often talk about the effect of the parents on the child, but it works both ways. A poorly child has an enormous impact on a parent, and therefore the parent is deserving of and will benefit from the appropriate support.

Treating young people with eating disorders

For a detailed approach to the treatment of child and teen eating disorders, please refer to Chapter 41 of *Acupuncture for Babies, Children and Teenagers* by Rebecca Avern.

Fifteen years ago, I would occasionally have a child with an eating disorder come to my clinic. Now, I have several at any one time. Some come to me after an inpatient stay in a psychiatric hospital, others are receiving psychological therapies whilst remaining at home with their families. Yet others are on a long waiting list for psychological help. This latter group are in the catch-22 situation of having been told they are "not yet ill enough" to jump to the front of the queue. Telling a young person with a restrictive eating disorder that they are "not ill enough" is tantamount to encouraging them to restrict their food intake even more.

There is so much that we, as practitioners of TEAMs, can do to help young people with eating disorders in terms of treating the underlying emotions, mitigating the physical damage and providing a space for them to explore and express whatever has caused the disordered eating (which is always the *biao* and never the *ben*). There are also some extra considerations that we should bear in mind.

We do not need to talk about food or weight

Providing that we know the young person is also being looked after by other healthcare professionals, we may be the one person in their lives who is not constantly grilling them about what they have eaten, what they haven't eaten and whether they are inducing vomiting and tracking their weight. Of course, we don't want this to be the elephant in the room, but relating to them as a person, rather than only "a person with an eating disorder" is healing in itself.

I find that young people with eating disorders really value being provided with a space to talk about how they feel, what makes them tick and what sparks joy in them. It can remind them that they are so much more than a person with an eating disorder.

Be mindful of your words

The mind of a young person struggling with disordered eating may interpret what is meant as an innocuous comment in a different way than it is meant. For example, simply saying, "You look well," may be interpreted as, "I must have put on weight." Some phrases we commonly use to describe what we are doing such as "nourishing blood" and treating "deficiency" or "excess" may be misconstrued. We should do our utmost to avoid saying anything that might feed the young person's destructive thoughts.

Adapt your questions during the intake

When working with young people with disordered eating, it is necessary to adapt the questions you ask during your intake. I usually omit asking about daily food intake and diet and may also omit asking questions about bowel habits. There are, of course, some young people who are far enough into their recovery for these areas not to be a problem. However, unless we are sure enough of that, it is wise to avoid them.

Be very wary of offering any dietary or nutritional advice

As practitioners of TEAMs, making dietary suggestions is a regular part of what we do. However, advising that a young person suffering from an eating disorder cuts out a particular food may feed into their restrictive eating. Suggesting that they include certain foods in their diet may provoke anxiety for them if they are not their "safe foods." This really feeds into the earlier point about generally not making your conversations with them about food any more than is necessary.

Think twice before prescribing herbs

There is no doubt that herbs can be very useful, especially for young people who have restricted their eating for a long time. However, if the young person is still in the grip of an eating disorder, it is possible that they may count any herbs you give them as part of their calorific intake for that day. So we need to be sure that the young person has reached a stage of recovery where this will not be the case before prescribing them herbs.

Be sure to gain informed consent before any form of palpation

Of course, we always need to gain consent before we palpate a child, but we should expect that this may be an especially tricky area for a young person who is struggling with their body image. As always, when working with young people, we need to be creative, and if we cannot get certain information we would usually get from abdominal palpation, there is normally another method we can use, for example, tongue diagnosis, taking the pulse or assessing color, sound and odor.

Finally, when treating any young person with an eating disorder, remember the words of the *Ling Shu* Chapter 8 that, "When one applies medical treatment, one must keep in mind first of all, the patient's spirit."[31] Although eating disorders affect the body, they are rooted in the spirit.

Treating young people who are self-harming

> For a detailed approach to the treatment of self-harm with acupuncture, please refer to Chapter 42 of *Acupuncture for Babies, Children and Teenagers* by Rebecca Avern.

If you treat young people, a minority of them will be self-harming or will have self-harmed previously. As with eating disorders, self-harm is the *biao* and not the *ben*, but we must nevertheless bear certain things in mind when we come across it.

Times to speak and times to stay quiet

If you go to take the pulse and, as you pull up the young person's sleeve, you notice cutting marks, it can be hard to know whether or not to mention what you have seen. There is no right or wrong answer to this. Each situation needs to be judged on its own merits. Many young people carry a lot of shame attached to their self-harm, and even when mentioned in the kindest of ways, it may trigger the shame. There are other times when it feels dishonest not to allude to the fact you have seen the young person's scars. In each case, a helpful question to ask yourself before deciding whether or not to speak is, "Do I think it is going to enhance or break rapport?"

If I decide to say something, it may be along the lines of, "I can see there has been a time when you have cut yourself. If you feel now or in the future that it would be helpful for you to share more about this, I have an open and non-judgmental ear. If you feel you'd rather not, that's fine too."

Avoiding certain areas of the body

I am sometimes informed by a parent before I see their child that the young person has cutting marks on a particular area of the body and wants reassurance I will not expose that part of the body. Of course, my answer to this is always that it is absolutely fine, although this can make pulse diagnosis tricky, as the most common place for cutting is the wrists. Not being able to needle certain parts of the body means we need to be creative about which points we use to fulfil our treatment principles. There are also times when things change as we go through the course of treatment and my therapeutic relationship with the young person deepens. They may have started out feeling a need to conceal but, over time, decide they do want to share.

Focus on feelings and not behavior

In a similar way to our treatment of young people struggling with disordered eating, we do not need to check in with the young person each time we see them about how often they have self-harmed. If we keep our focus on helping them to explore their feelings and treating them in a way which promotes emotional regulation, the need to self-harm will gradually lessen and fade.

Location is revealing

Where a young person cuts themselves may, in my experience, be significant. Although it would, of course, be unwise to rely on this alone to make a diagnosis, it can be added into the mix with all our other diagnostic clues. For example, is a young person who cuts along the Pericardium or Heart channel struggling with feelings related to the Fire phase, such as a lack of self-love or social anxiety? Or are cuts along the Spleen channel on the inner thigh or the Stomach channel on the abdomen a misguided attempt to alleviate feelings of worry, related to an Earth phase imbalance?

Be mindful of the young person's approach to acupuncture

On a few occasions over the years, I have been concerned about a child's relationship with acupuncture. One case stands out of a very troubled young boy of eight years old. He used to ask me incessantly if he could have more needles in a way that deeply concerned me. I felt that he viewed being needled as a form of self-punishment. It is highly unusual for an eight-year-old to want as many needles as possible, and it seemed as if he almost wanted the needles to be painful. In this case, referring him on to a practitioner of a different therapy felt like the right thing to do. Whenever you get a little voice of unease trying to tell you something is not quite right, I urge you to stop, reflect, listen and act on it.

Treating children who are neurodiverse

For a detailed approach to the treatment of difficulties associated with autism with acupuncture, please refer to Chapter 39 of *Acupuncture for Babies, Children and Teenagers* by Rebecca Avern.

A word about terminology

During this section, I use the terms "neurodiverse" and "neurotypical." I do this for ease, although I have reservations about it. The more we go along with the idea that there is such a thing as "typical" and "non-typical," the more we embed the idea of difference and separation. It also suggests that it is binary and there is a precise moment or place where a child is no longer neurotypical and becomes neurodiverse. The reality is that it is a spectrum. Unfortunately, I have not been able to find more suitable terminology, so please bear this in mind.

Statistics suggest that in the past 20 years, the number of children diagnosed with an autism spectrum disorder has risen from

1 in 150 to 1 in 36.[32] From my personal experience of working with children, I see more and more who have a diagnosis related to neurodiversity or who I suspect are neurodiverse. There is so much that we can do to make the lives of these young people easier and help them to thrive in a world which is often not geared towards their needs. We cannot, and arguably would not want to, take away their neurodiversity. But we can help to mitigate some of the challenges that often come with it, such as sleep disturbance, anxiety, difficulty with emotional regulation and various physical complaints.

Of course, neurodiverse is a wide umbrella, and every neurodiverse child will need something a little different, just as every neurotypical child will. Below I outline some general considerations to bear in mind when working with children who are on the autism spectrum or have other elements of neurodiversity.

The need for time

Some neurodiverse children may need more time than the majority of neurotypical children to feel relaxed and adjust to the environment of your clinic. Coming to your clinic for the first time, meeting you and potentially receiving treatment that is unfamiliar to them may induce a significant amount of stress. Neurodiverse children may lack an "ozone layer" of protection, so if we approach too quickly or too strongly, they may feel bombarded or invaded. Due to their thin, outer layer of *qi* (in Chinese medicine terms we could class this is a *wei-ying* imbalance), they may be highly attuned to the "vibes" and will pick up a lot more information than another child might. This takes time to make sense of and process.

So we should approach treatment cautiously and slowly, especially in the early stages. Below are a few suggestions of how to make the process for a neurodiverse child easier for them:

- Before the first appointment, suggest to the parent that they bring their child to your clinic a few times. Maybe they can sit in the waiting room a little, meet you when you come through to collect your next patient, perhaps come through to have a look at your treatment room. All of this will give the child a chance to orient themselves and feel more relaxed before the first session.

- During your sessions, it may be helpful to take the entire process of treatment really slowly. For example, a child may not feel comfortable with sticking out their tongue until they get to know you better. It may be wise to introduce one treatment method at a time and start with your least invasive. The key point is that you need to be constantly sensing what the child can manage. As soon as you feel they are retreating, you need to ease off.

Furthermore, a neurodivergent child will likely have an especially strong emotional memory. So if an experience feels uncomfortable, stressful or in some way not right, they will tend to retain a very strong memory of it. They are likely to then associate you and your clinic with that unpleasant emotional memory for a long time to come.

As Confucius wrote in the *Analects*:

> If a man is brusque in his movements, others will not co-operate. If he is agitated in his words, they awaken no echo in others. If he asks for something without having first established relations, it will not be given to him.[33]

Quami is on the autism spectrum. When I first met him, he had not been to school since before the Covid-19 pandemic, which was five years ago. He rarely left his home. His parents were desperate for him to have treatment but were really concerned about how they could get him to me. They were also concerned that Quami would not be able to manage bumping into other people in my clinic. So we made a plan.

First, Quami came to the gate of the clinic a few times and just hung out there. I popped out to see him and say hello a few times when he was there. Next, he bypassed my waiting room and came into my treatment room and had a look around a few times. We agreed that he could always bypass the waiting room (luckily, I also have a door directly from the outside into my treatment room). Third, we agreed that I would message his parents when my previous client had left, signally that Quami could come in from his car without bumping into anyone.

Quami's dad always messages me before a treatment with an update, as Quami hates any conversation to do with his health. So when he arrives, he just hops straight up onto the treatment table and I begin treatment.

This has worked really well, and I am happy to report that Quami loves his treatments and is benefitting from them.

Hypersensitivity to touch

Some neurodiverse children may be hypersensitive to touch. At home, they may dislike the sensation when their hair is brushed or the feel of certain clothes against their skin. Someone unexpectedly putting a hand on their shoulder may feel uncomfortable for them. Obviously, the vast majority of our treatment methods involve direct touch. Below are some suggestions of how we might approach touch on a child who is sensitive to it:

- For many neurodiverse children, it is not so much the touch that is difficult but the fact that it is unexpected. Making sure that you explain to a child before you perform any kind of physical contact is therefore important. I have also found that for many children, intentional touch such as pediatric *tui na* strokes can be very well tolerated, especially when I find the right degree of pressure. Sometimes, firmer, stronger touch is better received than very light touch.

- It can be helpful to make initial contact at the extremities, in particular the hands. This is often less threatening than being touched on the torso or the head. After all, the traditional "handshake" has for millennia been a way of two people introducing themselves to each other. I might begin my treatment by finding something I can do on the child's hand, and then, with their consent, gradually expand to the arm and maybe the lower leg. Again, it's a matter of sensing what the child can tolerate, going at their pace and being creative if you can't do your treatment on the part of the body you ideally would like.

When I had an initial phone call with Lyla's mum, she explained to me that Lyla struggles with any kind of touch. When I first saw Lyla, I made sure to ask for her consent before every step of the treatment. For example, I asked if it would be OK if I put my fingers on her wrist to feel her pulse. I began by using indirect moxa and a laser pen, which I hovered just above her skin. However, as Lyla became more relaxed with me, she allowed me to use press needles, direct moxa and some pediatric *tui na* on her head, which she said she found extremely relaxing. Lyla had her limits in terms of touch. She said that her abdomen and lower back were "out of bounds," for example. As long as I asked for her consent and very clearly explained before I did anything, she really enjoyed her treatments. Through the experience, she also learned that touch was not always something she found difficult but could even be something she enjoyed.

A difficulty with direct questions about health

Any child may struggle to answer questions about their health. But some neurodiverse children may struggle more than others. There are several possible reasons for this. One is that it is difficult for some neurodiverse children to connect with or make sense of what is going on in their bodies. In Chinese medicine terms, the *po* spirit is often not well housed in the *jing*, and therefore the child is not, to some degree, "in" their body. Another reason is that direct questions about health are often stressful for a neurodiverse child. They may worry that they cannot give you the "right" answer and can feel easily overwhelmed by any degree of questioning. For some children, it feels in some way stressful or anxiety-provoking to have to think about their health and their bodies.

As always, there are things that we can do to work around this, as suggested below:

- You may want to arrange with the parent that they give you an update before the appointment.

- Some children may not want to answer your questions themselves but are happy for their mum or dad to answer them for them.

- You may find it useful to have some emoji charts in your clinic which a child can pick out to indicate how they are feeling.

- One neurodiverse child I worked with really enjoyed writing down what she wanted to tell me rather than speaking. So she came to each appointment with a pre-written diary of her week. This is something that you might feel is worth suggesting to some children.

Challenges with emotional regulation

One of the greatest challenges for many neurodiverse children is to regulate their emotions. The same level of emotion in a neurodiverse child compared with a neurotypical one may feel very different. A neurodiverse child may experience the emotion as if it were a tidal wave overwhelming them, whereas for another child, the emotion may feel like a small, gentle wave. So, when we are working with neurodiverse children in our clinics, they will at times become overwhelmed by an emotion, whether that be anger, sadness or anxiety, for example.

Our aim is not to try to stop this from happening but to manage it as best we can when it does happen. There are two rules of thumb for this, which I outline below.

- Remain as calm, centered and grounded as you can in yourself. Do not meet fire with fire! As the practitioner, you need to be the *yin* to the child's *yang* in that moment of overwhelm. It comes down to not being afraid of intense emotional expression, allowing it to happen and knowing it will pass. Of course, there may be times when we need to put boundaries around certain behaviors and make sure we and our clinics remain safe. Separating emotion from behavior is the key.

- Avoid saying or doing anything that might induce feelings of shame in the child. Many children experience intense emotions of shame, guilt or regret in response to the original intense emotion. Showing them that we totally accept them, strong emotions and all, is healing for them.

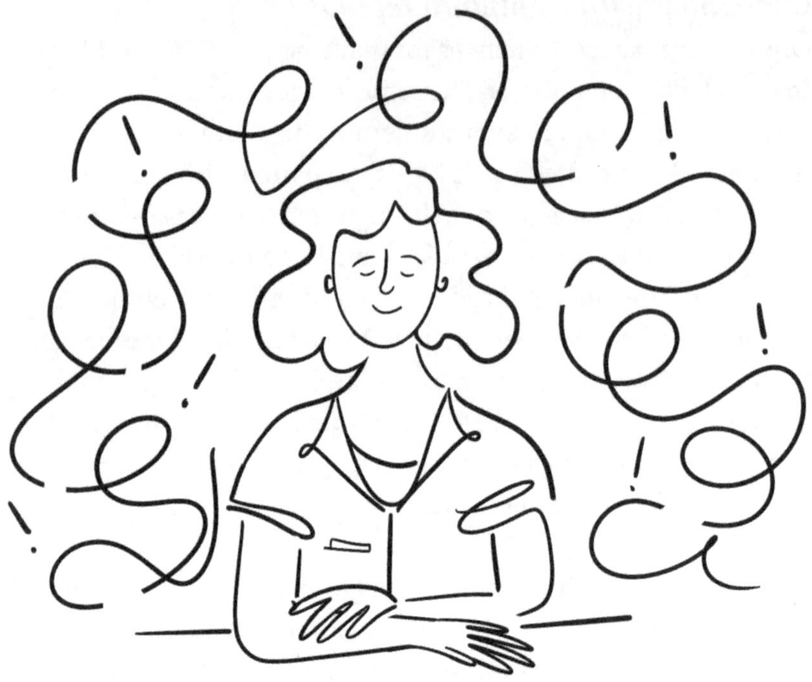

Managing expectations

Many societies are slowly but surely becoming more aware of the needs of neurodiverse people, and small changes are beginning to happen. For example, some cinemas have special showings for people with autism spectrum disorder who may find the usual volume painful. There is such a long way to go in this sphere, however, and sadly, neurodiverse children are currently expected to cope in a world which is not well attuned to their needs. For this reason, their challenges will not go away. We should expect that a neurodiverse child with anxiety will need more ongoing treatment than a neurotypical child, because the world they live in presents them with many challenges on a daily basis.

When I am working with neurodiverse children and their families, I suggest that we see each other regularly for however it long it takes for the child to feel really relaxed and comfortable coming to see me. Once that has been achieved, and we have also begun to see some improvements in the child's symptoms, then treatments can be spaced further apart. We will work towards finding a spacing that is enough to keep the child's symptoms at bay or at a manageable level and works for the family financially.

Masking

Masking involves hiding a discomfort or an emotion and can be an attempt to portray oneself as being more like a neurotypical child. It is common in neurodiverse children and can be either conscious or subconscious. In clinic, this often manifests as the child seemingly being absolutely fine with being needled, for example, whereas in reality they do not feel fine. As practitioners, it is important to be aware of this to ensure that we are genuinely providing the child with an enjoyable treatment experience.

Signs that a child may be masking include:

- avoiding eye contact or maintaining unnatural eye contact with you
- facial expressions and gestures that do not seem quite natural to you
- an over-compliant or extremely eager to please nature.

Every child will mask in a different way, but ultimately, as the practitioner, you need to trust your instincts. If you ever have a feeling of surprise that a child is saying yes to everything you are suggesting in terms of treatment, even though you have been told by the parent that they are hypersensitive to touch, then that child is highly likely to be masking. Check in with the child repeatedly about how they are finding the needles, the *shonishin* or whatever else you are doing. It can also be helpful to ask for their consent to use a particular treatment modality in a way that makes it easy for them to say no. For example, rather than saying, "I'd like to needle a point on your leg—is that OK?" you might say, "I could needle this point but am equally happy to use my laser pen—which would you prefer?"

Special interests

Many neurodiverse children have a particular subject or area of life in which they have huge interest and often knowledge, too. They often love to talk about this. I have learned so much about all sorts of obscure subjects from some of my neurodiverse children over the years. I find that when I show interest in this subject and invite the young person to talk about it, it really relaxes them. It also helps me to connect with them, and our rapport deepens. All of this means that the child generally finds it easier to have their treatment and the session goes smoothly.

Avoid making assumptions

Assumptions about people are rarely a good thing. We probably all have preconceptions about the nature of neurodiverse kids, as if they were all alike, which, of course, they are not. Many a time, people have said to me that an autistic child would never be able to tolerate acupuncture, for example. This is simply not true. When working with neurodiverse children, but really when working with *any* children, I urge you to put all preconceptions and assumptions to one side. That way, you will see the child as they really are and form a therapeutic relationship with them rather than a preconceived idea of them.

I have some neurodiverse clients who I use only my most gentle non-needle techniques on. I have others who are entirely happy with and actually enjoy needles. I have some who love to chat to me about how they are feeling and others who do not want to chat at all. Some are intrigued by acupuncture and Chinese medicine, and it has become an interest or even a passion for them.

There may be some neurodiverse children for whom your treatment simply does not feel right. That's OK! There will also be some young people on the extreme end of the autism spectrum who it is just not possible for you to treat. I have sadly had to decline treating a small handful of children over the years because I simply could not find a way to manage them in the treatment room and it did not feel right either for them or for me. However, for many neurodiverse children, your treatment will not only feel right but may also feel like one of the few things in their lives which help them to feel better. I urge you to welcome neurodiverse children into your clinic and to have the confidence that you and your treatment can be a positive force in their lives.

Summary

There are challenges involved with working with young people, and those challenges are greater when working with young people who have particular individual needs. Yet at the same time, these children are some of the most neglected, and they are badly in need of our help. I find that often it is when we meet our greatest challenges as a practitioner that we grow the most and, ultimately, gain the most rewards. So I encourage you, once again, to follow the words of the great Sūn Sī Miao and, "create a heart intent on relieving suffering. Then, even in the midst of the darkest fate, you will feel yourself blessed in multiple ways."[34]

Section 2

THE PRACTICALITIES OF WORKING WITH CHILDREN

CHAPTER 6

Delivering Treatment to Children

Delivering your treatment so children will accept it

Choosing the best treatment modalities is one thing but how we go about using them will play a large part in how well a child will accept them. Of course, every child will need a slightly different approach. The same child may need a different approach on a different day. They key, therefore, is to remain attuned to the child's needs and responses all the time. Beyond that, there are certain tips and tricks which I find useful.

Avoid surprises

When working with a verbal child, it is important and necessary to avoid "surprising" them with what you are doing. Most children do not take kindly to this. Doing something without their consent does not create trust and a feeling of safety. Children are especially susceptible to fright, which we want to avoid at all costs during treatment, as it causes dysregulation. Sūn Sī Miao stressed the importance of this when he said:

> Constantly beware of fright while rearing small children. Do not let them hear loud noises and, when holding them in your arms, be still and gentle. Do not let them be frightened or startled.

> Moreover, when there is thunder in the sky, plug the children's ears.[35]

So before delivering any treatment of any kind, prepare the child, demonstrate and/or explain so that they know what is coming.

Engagement versus distraction

Some children like to be involved in every stage of their treatment. They like to watch the needles being inserted, tell you when they feel *de qi*, press the buttons on "the beepy machine" and help you make sure their stickers are properly on. This is great, and if a child wants to be engaged in their treatment in this way, I encourage it. It can at times feel like a really strong need to be involved is bordering on a somewhat unhealthy need to control their environment, in order to allay an underlying anxiety. If this is the case, I see it as a good sign when, somewhere down the line, the child takes more of a back seat.

However, there are also children for whom it works best to be absorbed in or even distracted by something during the treatment. Having prepared and explained to them what we are going to do, they then relax more if they are chatting away to you or their parent, looking at a book or playing with a toy. Of course, there are also children who like to be engaged with some parts of the treatment and distracted at other times. We need to deliver our treatment in a way which works best for the child.

Being in sync

Treatment always goes with a flow when we are in sync with a child. *Su Wen* Chapter 14 explains that, "When doctor and patient are in a state of harmony, the illness will not linger or become terminal..."[36] From the moment we first see them, we need to begin to pick up on how the child is and what they need. There may be something about their body language, eyes or complexion which indicates they are feeling a certain way. If we respond to that and are there for them in the way they need, they will allow us to do much more than if we are not.

It might be helpful to understand more deeply this state of "being in sync" by looking at the Chinese term *dé*. It includes the characters for both "heart" and "brain." Wilms translates this term as "heart-sounding."[37] To know what a child needs and to get in the flow with them means employing our senses as much as our thinking capacity. I love the term "heart-sounding" because to me it suggests the idea of a rhythm and a beat, and we need to strive to find a rhythm in the way we connect to a child. It's all very well being a virtuoso violinist, but unless you are aware of, listen to and respond to the other players in the orchestra, your virtuosity will have a limited impact. The same goes for us as practitioners. Our skills are limited by the degree to which we can tune in to every child we treat.

In practical terms, this means noticing the little things and accommodating them. If a child arrives looking cold, tired and miserable after a day at school, it might work best to get them straight onto the treatment table (if that's where they usually have their treatment) and snuggle them up in a blanket rather than having them sit on a chair or beanbag first. That way, they can immediately relax and get comfortable rather than us having to ask them to move from beanbag to treatment table during the session. If a child is prone towards hyperactivity, I often ask the parent to update me on how they have been prior to the session so I can just get treating as quickly as possible before they start to feel constrained. If I know a certain child can be sensitive to any kind of touch or treatment, I might work really hard to get them talking about something that fires them up so they almost do not notice that they are receiving a treatment. These little details help us to "heart-sound" with the child.

Positioning the child

Where a child sits can make a big difference to how relaxed they feel. For a young child, we might carry out their treatment with them sitting on a parent's lap. Sometimes, I have the parent on the treatment table with the child sitting on top of them. Some children like to have their treatment on a beanbag or even sitting under the treatment table whilst playing with a toy. I have treated some children in my waiting room when they have a resistance to walking through to the treatment room.

Whilst flexibility on the practitioner's behalf is key, it is also acceptable to have limits! It is one thing to agree to carry out a child's treatment on the beanbag (even though it may not be ideal) when they are obviously feeling fearful and genuinely nervous of getting on the treatment table. It is another when they are simply messing around and trying to annoy either their parent or us.

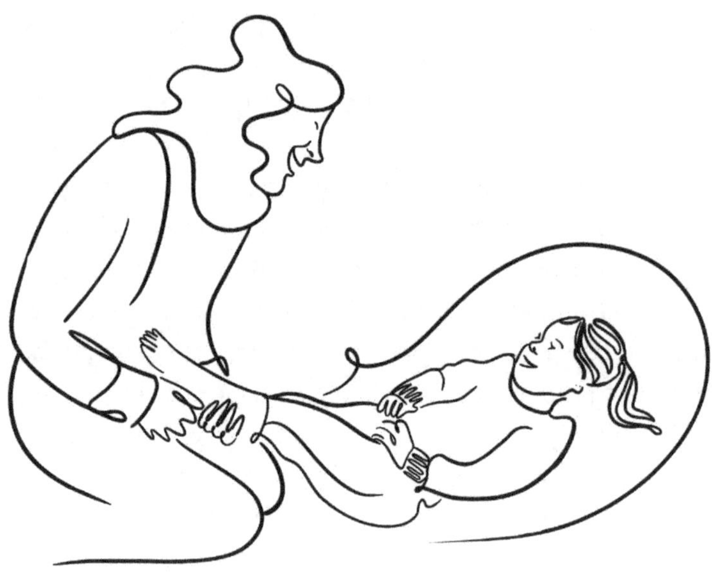

Toys and books

Every pediatric clinic must have a good selection of toys and books. I keep mine in the waiting room so children see them immediately when they arrive, signaling to them that this is a child-friendly place. They can then choose one or two to bring through to the treatment room. Having a child play with a toy or look at a book can be relaxing and can entertain them while we carry out their treatment. Whilst some children are able to relax into their treatment, space out and switch off, many will find lying or sitting still for 10 or 20 minutes difficult. Many children are habituated to always being stimulated. Having something to do, therefore, actually feels more relaxing to them than not doing anything. I sometimes find that parents tell their children to relax while they are having their treatment. First, this is unrealistic for some children and also unnecessary. Second, being told to relax is deeply unrelaxing!

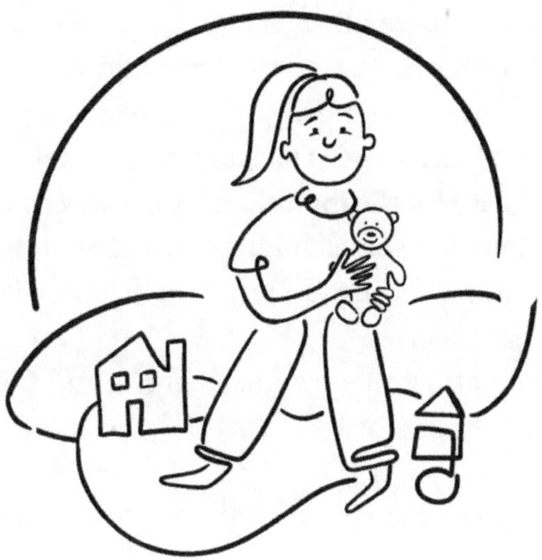

However, there are limits that need to be set around the use of toys. Having one or two small toys on the treatment table may work well. More than that may be a hindrance. I find it helpful to have some general protocols to which I ask children to adhere. For example, they can choose two small toys to take to the table with them and play with anything else after the treatment in the waiting room (if the parent has time).

In terms of books, an older child may bring a book with them which they are currently reading, whilst I have a selection of books for younger children already in my clinic. However, the best solution for books for children right up to the pre-teen years (and sometimes beyond) is to have a collection of "search and find" books, such as *Where's Waldo?*.* These type of books can keep children engaged for long periods of time whilst simply using their visual acuity rather than taxing their Spleen *qi*.

Screens

Whether we like it or not, children will come to the clinic with screens, ask for their parent's phone during the treatment and sometimes even expect us to have a device they can use whilst having their treatment. The question of what we do about this and whether or not we allow screens during treatments is a potent one. When I first started treating children, I held a strong view that I would *never* allow the use of screens in my treatment room. With time and experience, my view softened. I realized that there is a place for the intentional use of screens in the pediatric clinic. There are some children for whom doing a screen-based activity relieves their anxiety to an extent that they then allow us to treat them.

When we do allow the use of screens, I find the following limits helpful:

- Watching a cartoon or a favorite show on a screen is acceptable. Playing a fast-moving and agitating game is not.
- Children tend to love looking at pictures of themselves! One of the most benign screen-based activities is for a child to look through the Photos app on a parent's phone, if the parent agrees to this of course.
- Before being given the device, I ask the child to agree to certain things. For example, they can use it on the basis that I am then allowed to deliver the treatment that they have agreed to. Or they can use a device for a certain part of

* In the UK, Waldo is called Wally!

> the treatment. I always ask them to agree to put the device down near the end of the treatment. This is so I can engage with them before they leave. I really do *not* feel comfortable with a child walking away from my treatment room still engrossed in whatever they are doing on their screen.

I ensure that the use of a device does not become a bargaining tool for the child. If I sense a child is playing up in order to be allowed to use a device, I try my best not to collude. It has to be our decision whether or not we allow a child the use of a device, rather than something we get coerced into. Being on a screen has a place when we decide that it will help a child to be able to receive the treatment they need.

Here are some useful props that it might be handy to keep in your clinic:

- A selection of books for all ages.
- Some cuddly toys.
- A few carefully chosen toys.
- Some puzzles.
- A few fidget toys.
- A small bubble machine—brilliant for entertaining babies and toddlers.
- Colored salt timers (for a child to hold and let you know when the time is up).

- An eyeliner pencil—drawing little pictures or marking where you are going to put a needle is a fun icebreaker!
- Stickers—my clinic is called The Panda Clinic; every child who visits is offered a panda sticker when they leave.
- Emoji charts—to help a child identify what they may be feeling.

How to needle a child

If children were blasé about needles, our work would be entirely transformed. Sadly, the vast majority of children are far from relaxed on this matter. It is therefore a central part of our work to find our way around this. Becoming adept at using many of the non-needle techniques available to us is the subject of Chapters 7 and 8. Another key aspect of this, however, is learning how to prepare children for needling and to actually needle them in an acceptable way.

I have a suspicion, confirmed by colleagues who were treating children a couple of decades before I was, that there are more children today who are resistant to the idea and reality of needles than in previous generations. There are several possible reasons for this. The nervous systems of many children today are over-stimulated and turned up a notch compared with children of decades ago. Children today also receive many more vaccinations, so they often come to us with negative connotations of needles already. Children born in the last decade or so are more likely to have been raised to speak their mind about what they do and don't want (which, of course, is a good thing!).

There are, of course, differences between children. I practice in a small city, and I have noticed that children who come to see me from villages or small towns in the countryside are, on the whole, more relaxed about needles than children who live in the city. City kids often have a more tense and wired system, which can make them more sensitive to any kind of discomfort. Babies up to the age of approximately 18 months are usually entirely happy to be needled and often smile and look rather blissed out and spacey during the needling. Phlegmy children are often the most nonchalant about needling; deficient and sensitive children are often the most anxious about it.

There are many trends. These are all simply that, however—just trends. There are always exceptions, and it is rarely helpful for us to make assumptions based on the age and type of child about whether or not they will tolerate needles. I have been amazed by some of the children I would have least expected to tolerate needles actually enjoying them and vice versa.

I have some rules of thumb I follow which help me to decide whether using needles is the best course of action or not:

- If the parent reports, or I suspect, that the child will worry about the needles between appointments, I take needling out of the equation. We really do not want a child worrying all week about their next session, as the worry is likely to be counterproductive. Furthermore, we want the child to have largely positive feelings about their acupuncture sessions.

- Learn to distinguish between genuine fear and "faux fear," which may actually be an attempt to get some attention from Mum or to negotiate a reward (I am astounded by the negotiation skills of even very young children, most of whom I assume will go far in life if they are so adept at getting what they want at this age). The difference between genuine fear and "faux fear" is not usually hard to spot. In the presence of genuine fear, you will most likely respond with the knowledge that this is not the time to push it. In the presence of faux fear, you may find your response is more one of irritation!

- I do not mind if a child feels momentary discomfort when being needled but is absolutely fine shortly afterwards. Children do not have to really enjoy being needled (although some do), but if the upset is either intense or long, it will probably outweigh any benefits of the treatment.

General guidelines for needling a child

Rapport comes first

As always, rapport is everything in the treatment of children, and needling a child with whom we have good rapport is an entirely different experience to needling a child with whom we don't have good rapport. I recommend introducing needles only once you feel that you have made a connection with the child and that they trust you and feel relaxed. It may be that this is in the first session. Or it may not be until session 6 or session 20.

Honesty is the best policy

I am often asked whether or not I call a needle a needle with children. In my opinion, honesty is the best policy, and once a child has reached an age where we can have this kind of conversation, I absolutely call a needle a needle. However, I will show them the needle, let them hold a needle (in its guide tube), demonstrate needling on myself or the parent and illustrate to them that my needles are very different to the needles they have had at the doctors. I often show them a picture of an acupuncture needle alongside a hypodermic needle to illustrate the fact that my needles are incredibly fine.

I want to create a relationship of trust with a child. Furthermore, children are astute. If you trick them, you lose their trust, most likely forever.

Seamlessly interweave your needling into the treatment

Needling is just one part of a long "conversation" that you have with a child, which will also include chatting, palpating, using other techniques, having fun, etc. Try to avoid building up to the moment of needling as if it were a pinnacle. Think of it, and present it, as just one of the things that is going to happen during the session which is of no more or less importance than any of the other parts.

Timing is everything

Timing is very much related to rapport. Pushing needling on a child too early on in the process and them not liking it may mean they never let you try again. Waiting until they are ready to give it a go allows the child to feel they have some agency in the situation. I treat children with needles now who were strongly opposed to the idea of ever trying them when I first met them. At some stage during their treatment, they have often asked me if they can try them rather than me suggesting it to them. Kids feel so proud of themselves when they decide to give it a go and realize it's fine.

Examine your own fears or hesitation

One of the most powerful things you can do to successfully needle a child is to make sure you are in the best mindset possible. If you feel fearful about causing them pain, hesitant about whether it's the right course of action or frustrated because you just want to get on with it, the child will pick this up and they will resist you needling them. Some children will also resist if they feel a desperation in you to do it. Fortunately, there are *always* alternatives, so we can be genuinely relaxed about whether the child accepts needles or not.

The process of needling a child

Prepare the parent

Some parents who bring their child to you will have received acupuncture themselves and may be very relaxed about you needling their child. Others will want reassurance that their child will not find the experience painful. The easiest way to provide this is to needle the parent. I will needle them, making sure to avoid an acupuncture point (without having made a diagnosis, I do not want to needle a point or channel that is not indicated for them). This reassures the parent and they can then reassure the child about what they felt, so this is a win-win situation!

Prepare the child

How you prepare a child will depend very much on their age and personality.

The important aspects to describe are exactly what the process will be (whether you will leave the needle in or take it straight out, what you want them to do, etc.). As mentioned above, I often demonstrate on the parent or myself (or a cuddly toy!).

Prepare yourself

Ling Shu Chapter 9 tells us:

> Prior to needling a practitioner should retire to a quiet place and commune with his spirit with doors and windows shut. The doctor's *hun* and *po* must not be scattered, his mind must be focused, and his essence undivided. Undistracted by human sounds, he must marshal his essence, concentrate his mind and direct his will entirely towards needling.[38]

Whilst it may rarely be possible for us to "retire to a quiet place" before we needle each child, the point is that we need to create an internal state as if we were able to afford that luxury. The more focused and calm we are, the better the needling will go.

Here is an example of a narrative I might use with a child who is around the age of eight when I first needle them: "So, I'm going to insert the needle here on your leg, and I want you to keep your leg as floppy and relaxed as you can. First,

I will rest this tube on your skin, and then I will ask you to take a deep breath in. As you breathe out, I will gently tap the needle. I'm then going to ask you to say the magic words, 'Bippety bippety bop,' and by the time you've said that, I will have taken the needle out. Do you have any questions before we give it a go?"

Prepare the point

I find it helpful to gently rub the skin over the point I intend to needle. This disperses the *qi* at the surface, lessening the chances of the child feeling an intense sensation when I insert the needle.

The moment of insertion

Up until the age of around nine (by which time, they are far too cool for this), I ask the child to help me make the magic work. This involves saying the magic words, "Bippety bippety bop." The purpose of the magic words is to distract the child from the sensation of the needle (as well as them actually making the magic happen, of course!). They are fun words to say, and this involves the child so they do not feel like something is merely being done to them.

I also find it helpful to make sound effects as I needle. So just before I insert the needle, I will often say, "Tap tap tap tap," so that the child is tuned in to what I am saying rather than focusing on where I am putting the needle.

In the midst of all these considerations, the skill lies in remembering that: "The mind of the physician and the mind of the patient should be level, in harmony following the movements of the needle."[39]

Some other considerations

You will need to adapt how you needle with almost every child you see. With most children, I ask them to take a deep breath in and I insert the needle on the out breath. However, I have one child who insists that instead of saying, "Breathe in," I say, "3, 2, 1," before I needle her. Some children will feel more relaxed if they are looking at what you are doing, whilst others prefer to be looking at a book or holding their parent's hand. The key is to find out what works for each child.

Another aspect to be aware of is the build-up to needling. Some children become more anxious if they have time to think about it. So, whilst I would never recommend needling a child without letting them know that is what you are going to do, with some it works best to let them know and then immediately do it. On the other hand, some children benefit from having a little more time in the lead up to needling to prepare themselves. The more you are tuned in to the child, the better you will be able to intuit what the best approach is going to be.

Doing too much

One of the most common mistakes to make when treating children is to do too much. This may happen because the practitioner approaches the treatment in the same way they would for an adult or because they fear the parent's disapproval if their treatment has been minimal. As soon as you sense a shift in the *qi* of the child, stop! Try to stay connected with your professional confidence. It is more likely that you are doubting yourself than that the parent is doubting you.

Prioritizing "getting your treatment done" rather than making it enjoyable

Remember to think long term. If you push more treatment on a child than they are ready to accept, they may never come back. Rapport should *always* come first. Furthermore, parents generally understand this. They do not want their child to feel anxious or uncomfortable.

Lack of preparation and explanation

As we are so familiar with our medicine and its techniques, it is easy to forget that a lot of what we do is totally foreign to many of the children we see. I have seen kids who think there is something in my needles that I am injecting into them or who see me lighting a moxa stick and assume I am going to burn them. Always err on the side of overexplaining.

Forgetting to pay attention to the little things

Children notice and will remember how you greet them, how you say goodbye to them, whether or not you check they are comfortable and whether you keep your focus on them while you are treating them or get sidetracked by a parent or sibling. The little things are the big things. Pay attention to them.

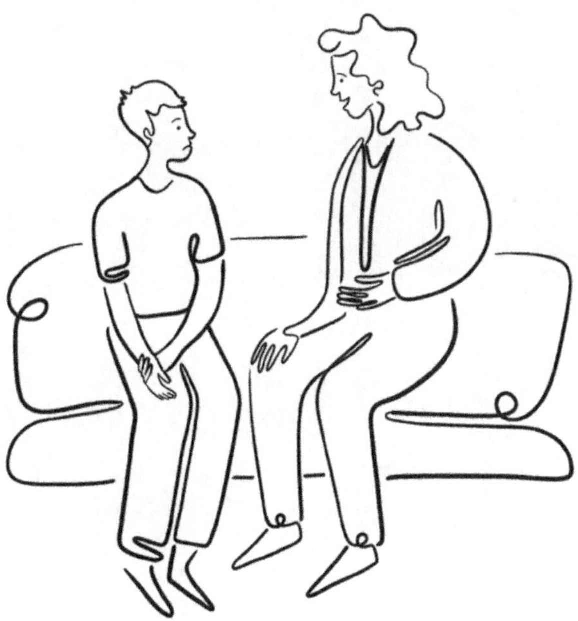

Summary

Being skilled at delivering your treatment is one of the key aspects that sets pediatrics apart from the treatment of adults.

It requires endless patience, "heart-sounding," sensitivity, tact and flexibility. However, at the root of it all is, of course, our relationship with the child. Without this, we have nothing. The physician Abraham Verghese sums this up beautifully when he says:

> We learn from medicine everywhere that it is, at its heart, a human endeavor, requiring good science but also a limitless curiosity and interest in your fellow human being, and that the physician-patient relationship is key; all else follows from it.[40]

Chapter 7

Traditional Methods of Treating Children

If we had to put our fingers on one, huge, massive, enormous barrier to all children receiving acupuncture, it would be the fact that it involves needles. Even those parents who have acupuncture themselves, and who believe in the power of TEAMs, often have the worry that their children will not tolerate needles. When I tell people I am a pediatric acupuncturist, a common response is, "How on earth do you do acupuncture on children?"

There are two key points to make in response to this question:

- Acupuncture needles do not need to be painful at all (see Chapter 6).
- Acupuncture does not need to involve the insertion of needles.

In this chapter, we will look at traditional alternatives to needles, and their advantages and disadvantages, and how to choose the best modality for each child. Some of these methods were developed specifically to treat children, i.e., pediatric *tui na* and *shonishin*. Others were not but can be adapted to use with children.

It is, of course, not possible to learn some of the practical techniques described below from a book. Many of the techniques described are taught in acupuncture undergraduate courses. Where this is not the case, I will indicate for each technique what I believe is the best way to become proficient at it.

Pediatric *tui na*

What is it?

Pediatric *tui na* (*xiao er tui na*) is a complete system of treatment in itself. The first mention of it was in Ming dynasty texts, although scholars believe it was used before this.

Pediatric *tui na* uses some acupuncture points but mainly uses areas or lines on the body, reflecting the fact that the channel system is not fully developed in young children. It gains its power from repetition of certain movements rather than from force. So it is gentle, relatively easy to do and, more importantly, extremely powerful in its therapeutic effect.

What age group can you use it with?

Opinions differ on this question. After around a decade of using it daily in my practice, I have come to the following conclusions:

- The moves on the hand are only really useful up until the age of seven or eight but are most effective up to around the age of five.
- The moves on the head, front and back torso can be used and are effective right into the teenage years.
- Over the age of seven or eight, pediatric *tui na* is better when combined with other modalities.

What are its main strengths?

There are several major benefits but the most outstanding is its extraordinary effectiveness. I have treated children with serious health problems with *tui na* alone many times and seen incredible results. I believe this is because it's possible to create a routine which directly addresses the pathologies of each child. Furthermore, because it uses lines and areas rather than points, it is perfectly suited to the developmental stage of a young child.

Its other great strength is how well tolerated it is. There is something about the repetition of the movements that often sends children into a deeply relaxed state. The beneficial effects of touch are now well documented. Positive touch helps to bring about a parasympathetic state, promote healthy brain development and reduce anxiety and pain, and it also helps children to fully inhabit their bodies and feel comfortable in them. When we perform pediatric *tui na*, children receive all these benefits on top of the fact that we are using it to address their particular pathologies. This is a powerful combination!

Another benefit of pediatric *tui na* is that it uses the same pattern differentiation system as Traditional Chinese Medicine (TCM) acupuncture. So practitioners who are used to diagnosing patterns according to *zangfu* and pathogen pathologies can make their diagnosis in the way they are used to. They treat as they would with acupuncture, but with *tui na* instead. In particular, pediatric *tui na* has the power to treat the following pathologies:

- Deficiency of any *zang* organ
- Deficiencies of *qi*, *yin* and *yang*
- Phlegm
- Heat
- Rebellious *qi*
- Accumulation Disorder
- *Shen* disharmonies.

Although adjuvants, such as powder or oil, can be used, most of the time it is sufficient to do it without. A typical routine may take anywhere between approximately four to ten minutes.

Lastly, *tui na* can easily be taught to parents to do each day at home. This means the child will get better more quickly but also that the parent will feel empowered to help their child. It can be nothing short of excruciating for a parent to feel they cannot help ease their child's suffering.

What are its main weaknesses?

There is a certain proportion of children who struggle to tolerate pediatric *tui na*. This may be because they find it difficult to stay still for long enough or are resistant to touch. Having said this, some children who can't tolerate some types of touch accept the repetitive, intentional touch of *tui na* readily. So it is always worth trying. Similarly, even extremely wriggly or hyperactive children can sometimes relax into a *tui na* treatment when approached in the right way (see the following top tips!).

The other main limitation of pediatric *tui na* is that the therapeutic areas on the hand are less potent past the ages of seven or eight.

Top tips when performing pediatric tui na

- Summon your *yi*. Just because you are using your hands, rather than needles, does not mean that intention is any less important. On the contrary, you should be entirely clear about why you are doing every move you choose to do and how it benefits your therapeutic aims for that child.

- Summon your *zhi*. Most pediatric *tui na* moves are done for approximately one minute. One minute is a long time to be stroking a child's thumb or kneading a point on the bottom of their foot, for example. Moreover, completing a whole routine which comprises several different moves requires commitment and staying power.

- Many children will get "into the zone" and space out while you treat them with pediatric *tui na*. For those who don't, you will need to find ways to keep them engaged in the treatment. I have found the following useful:
  - Make sound effects as you do the moves.
  - Use colored salt timers that the child holds.
  - Keep a small bubble machine in your clinic and ask the parent to use it while you treat their child.
  - With an older child, get them talking about a subject that interests them.

- Be prepared to move with the child. It's not realistic to expect all children to be able to stay in the same place for the length of the routine. Moving with them will increase the chances of you carrying out the treatment successfully, as opposed to trying to constrain them.

- With parents, refer to pediatric *tui na* as "Chinese medical massage."

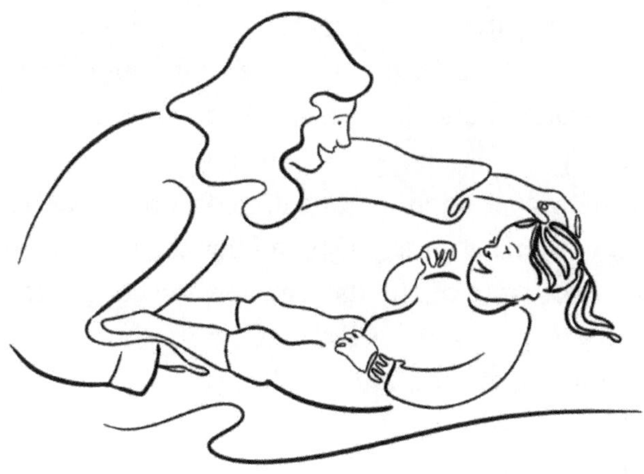

Teaching pediatric tui na to parents

The more thoroughly you teach a parent to perform *tui na*, the more likely they are to do it on their child at home. Below I set out the process I use to teach parents, which I have honed over the years.

1. Ensure that you allow sufficient time during an appointment rather than doing it in a rushed five minutes at the end. I tend to allow around 20 minutes.

2. Explain to the parent that you are teaching them Chinese medical massage which is specific to their child. I feel it's important to use the word "medical" so that we make it clear it is not simply the kind of massage you might do to help somebody relax. It's also necessary that they understand this is specific to this one child and would not be appropriate for another of their children.

3. Talk through the basic principles and back this up by giving the parent a sheet they can refer to that outlines what you have explained. These basic principles are as follows:

   - Each move should be done for approximately one to two minutes.
   - Classically, the moves on the limbs should be done on the right-hand side on a girl and the left-hand side on a boy.
   - The moves should all be done in one sequence, i.e., all together rather than spread out through the day.
   - Find a time of the day that best suits the family and when you are most likely to do it reliably. Before bedtime is good for many children, as the *tui na* will often help to promote sleep.
   - Pause doing the *tui na* if your child gets an acute illness, such as a cold or a gastric bug.

How to learn pediatric *tui na*

- *Acupuncture for Babies, Children and Teenagers* by Rebecca Avern includes an entire chapter on pediatric *tui na*, including illustrations, explanations and instructions for every *tui na* move.
- Hub of Pediatric Acupuncture (https://practitioner.pediatricacupuncture.org) members have access to professional videos of every pediatric *tui na* move, together with indications and clinical tips.
- If possible, find a two-day course in your area taught by someone knowledgeable and experienced in pediatric *tui na*.

Channel and point massage

What is it?

Channel and point massage is simply massage, or acupressure, on the acupuncture channels or parts of channels. It is a simplified version of *shiatsu* or *anma*.

What age group can you use it with?

Channel or point massage can be used on babies right through to teenagers. Just be sure not to massage over open fontanelles on young babies.

What are its main strengths?

Channel or point massage is an effective and well-tolerated way to help promote the flow of *qi* in a channel or stimulate or disperse a point. It is diagnostic as well as therapeutic. As we massage, we can feel for areas of particular flaccidity, blockages or changes of temperature.

Here are some of the ways I most commonly use channel or point massage in clinic:

- Massaging up the Spleen channel and down the Stomach channel on the lower leg. Considering that the Earth organs in nearly all young children are under strain, this is a great health prevention massage which can also be taught to parents.

- Massaging along the *du mai*, the Bladder and Gallbladder channels on the top of the head, from front to back. This is an excellent way to promote the circulation of *qi* and blood in the channels of the head, a pattern often found in children who have had a difficult birth, caesarean birth or forceps delivery.

- Massaging the *san jiao* channel together with some Gallbladder and Small Intestine points around the ear. Promoting the flow of *qi* in these channels which encircle the ear is useful in cases of glue ear and hypersensitivity to noise.

- Using acupressure on a particular point or pair of points when needles, moxa or other methods will not be tolerated or are not available.

What are its main weaknesses?

Children who have a lot of stagnation in the channel or area you want to massage may find it uncomfortable and difficult to tolerate. This in itself is a sign of stagnation.

Top tips when performing channel and point massage

- If the massage is uncomfortable, it is a sign that it needs to be done! I would first use a distraction technique such as asking the parent to look at a book with the child to see if they can tolerate it for a while. If this does not work, it's a matter of building it up little by little. The more you are able to do it, the more the child will tolerate it as the *qi* and blood start to move. This is one of the few situations where I recommend the parent carrying out the massage while the child is asleep, just until it is possible to do it when they are awake.

- When using channel massage on the head in particular, when you come across an area that feels hard or knotty, stay on it and do some vigorous rubbing for a few seconds to disperse the stagnation.

- Intention is just as important when using your hands as it is when using a needle. You will be more effective when your full intention is behind what you are doing for the duration.

Shonishin

What is it?

Shonishin is a Japanese term which can be roughly translated as "children's needle." It originated in Japan in the 17th century. *Shonishin* does not involve inserting needles but uses various tools on the surface of the skin. The tools are stroked, tapped or scraped, for example, depending on what therapeutic effect is desired. Just as with all aspect of TEAMs, there are many different styles and schools of *shonishin*.

What age group can you use it with?

Shonishin can be used with any age group, starting from premature babies and going upwards. When used on children from the age of approximately seven or eight upwards, I usually combine it with some of the other methods outlined in this book.

What are its main strengths?

Shonishin is extremely gentle and extremely quick to perform, both of which are beneficial when treating children. *Shonishin* can be used in the treatment of most conditions. Here are some situations when I tend to use it the most:

- In pre-term babies who are not "ill" as such but who may be struggling to make the transition to life outside the womb; this is because they were not quite developmentally ready to do so.

- In very small babies, with whom needling is not normally necessary and for whom it can feel counterintuitive to needle because of their fragility.

- In babies who are unsettled, unhappy or not feeding properly.

- At the beginning of a treatment with a child of any age as a way of helping them to relax before needling.

- There is a non-pattern-based *shonishin* treatment which can be done on most children without having previously made a diagnosis, as a way of "settling" the *qi* and calming the nervous system.

- In a child who has sensory processing issues, particularly ones related to tactility. *Shonishin* may help balance and normalize the sensations these children feel from their environment and in their bodies.

- In any child who has a pathology related to counterflow *qi* (*ni qi*) rising up to the head.
- In babies with KISS* syndrome.

What are its main weaknesses?

Shonishin is a wonderful form of treatment, but it has its limits. In my opinion, there are some conditions which only acupuncture can cure. *Shonishin* supports healthy growth and development and can be used in the treatment of common childhood ailments, but for more complex situations, it may not be enough on its own.

Top tips when performing shonishin

- A *shonishin* treatment can take as little as a couple of minutes and it can look to the untrained eye as if we have barely done anything at all. It takes some confidence to stop when we have done enough. It is important not to unnecessarily add in something extra because we are worried about being perceived as having barely done anything. I urge you to learn to sit with the discomfort you may feel in this situation rather than do more for the sake of it, which rarely has a good therapeutic outcome.
- Whenever we treat children, we need to be "in the zone" and in a "*qi* bubble" with them in order to be really effective. This is especially the case with *shonishin*. It is essentially a palpatory method of treatment, so we need to be really tuned in to the child's *qi* and their body in order to do it well.

---

* KISS stands for "Kinematic Imbalance due to Suboccipital Strain."

How to learn *shonishin*

I highly recommend any practitioner who would like to include this form of treatment in their practice to attend a practical course with an experienced *shonishin* practitioner. It is very much a palpation-based method of treatment in that how we do it is based on what we feel as we do it. Therefore, it is ideally learned in practical classes.

Please see the "Further resources" section for details of the two key books on *shonishin* currently available in English.

Moxibustion

What is it?

Moxibustion is a technique widely used in TEAMs, involving the burning of dried mugwort on acupuncture points, along channels or over areas of the body.

What age group can you use it with?

Moxibustion can be used in one form or another with children of every age. I tend to use different types of moxa on different age groups, outlined here.

Tiger warmer

This is one of the most gentle ways of using moxa, so I tend to use this method often on very young children. A tiger warmer is a metal moxa holder. A small, slow-burning lit moxa stick is placed inside the holder, and the end of the holder heats up. This warm end can be held on an acupuncture point, channel or over an area with a tissue between it and the skin to lessen the intensity of the heat.

Indirect moxa

Indirect moxa involves holding a moxa stick (or pole) over a point, channel or area without the moxa coming into direct contact with the skin. The stick is often "pecked" (i.e., lifted up and down). It has a slightly stronger effect than the tiger warmer. I tend to use indirect moxa on children from the age of approximately three upwards.

Direct moxa

Direct moxa involves burning small cones of loose moxa over acupuncture points. The cones are placed over a small amount of *shiunko* (purple mountain) moxa cream, and the top of the cone is lit with a Japanese incense stick. The cone is removed either when the child begins to feel the warmth, or when it has burned 80% of the way down, whichever happens first. This action is then repeated several times on the same point.

Direct moxa involves a child needing to stay still. Some children may also find they get a little concerned about the idea of lit moxa coming so close to their skin. For these reasons, I tend to use direct moxa from the age of approximately seven upwards, although the maturity of the child is more important than their age.

Stick-on moxa

Stick-on or adhesive moxa are mini pieces of a moxa roll attached to a sticker which can be placed on acupuncture points. Both smoky and smokeless versions are available, as well as "light" and "intense" versions. It can be used instead of either direct moxa or indirect moxa on an acupuncture point.

Electric moxa

Electric moxa machines are a relatively new invention. They may cost between $500 and $1000. They are pen-like machines which emit red, infrared and far infrared light at the same spectrum width and distribution as the burning of artemisia. They can be held just above an acupuncture point, or any part of the body, or they can touch the skin when used with a concentrator. Therefore, they can be used in place of any of the moxa types already described.

Electric moxa can be used on any child of any age.

What are its main strengths?

Moxa is a wonderful alternative to needling when we want to tonify an organ. Small amounts of moxa are strengthening rather than warming. There are multiple uses of moxa, including the following:

- Moxa is a great alternative to a needle when we want to tonify an organ.
- Moxa is also a very efficient way of nourishing blood and even *yin*.
- Moxa can be used to draw heat from one place in the body to another. Like attracts like, so using moxa on the foot, for example, can attract floating heat in the upper part of the body back down.
- Moxa (especially a tiger warmer) can be used to create movement and break down thick phlegm in the form of hard lymph nodes.

Many children find the use of moxa, especially on the lower part of the body, extremely relaxing and will ask for it again once they have experienced it for the first time.

What are its main weaknesses?

The main weakness is really more of a caution. There are inherent risks involved with using fire around young children. The practitioner needs to make a judgment with each child and in each situation as to whether or not it is sensible to use moxa.

Top tips when using moxa

- **For all types of moxibustion**: It is of paramount importance to always put safety first when using moxa around children. We must use moxa with extreme care, making sure to watch out for moving limbs and sudden movements that children are prone to make.

- **Demonstrate how you are going to use moxa on yourself or a parent before using it on a child**.

- **Be careful with your language**: Make it quite clear there are not going to be any flames involved and that the lit moxa will never come directly into contact with the child's skin.*

- **Tiger warmer**: Place a tissue between the warm end of the tiger warmer and the skin to lessen the heat sensation for the child.

- **Indirect moxa**: Unless you are using smokeless moxa, pole moxa can create a lot of smoke in the room. This can aggravate the chest in some children with asthma and respiratory conditions. I tend not to use this type of moxa around babies either, unless the room is extremely well ventilated.

- **Direct moxa**: When treating adults, it is common practice to leave the moxa cone in place until the patient says it feels too warm. The sting of heat that may be felt can be too strong and sudden for children. Remember, moxa is of therapeutic value as long as the moxa cone burns down

---

* I once treated a child who had previously seen another practitioner. They became very nervous when I began explaining the moxa process. It turned out that the previous practitioner had said they were going to "light bonfires on their skin" and they had never quite recovered from this!

at least 80% of the way. This means we can effectively use this type of moxa without the child needing to feel an uncomfortable heat sensation.

- **Indirect moxa**: It is essential to make sure that you frequently tap the end of the moxa pole to release the ash. Even a speck of ash falling on the child's skin may be enough to put them off ever trying it again.

- **Electric moxa and indirect moxa**: On a child who is too young to be able to tell you what they are feeling, place a finger either side of the point over which you are holding it. As you warm up the point, slide your fingers over it so that you can judge the degree to which it is heating up.

Table 7.1 summarizes the different types of moxa that can be used with children, the age group they can be used on and their strengths and weaknesses.

Table 7.1 Different types of moxa and their uses

Type of moxa	Age group	Strengths	Weaknesses
Tiger warmer	Any, but especially babies and toddlers	Very low dose, gentle moxa Does not produce much smoke	The end of the tiger warmer can get quite hot quite quickly
Indirect moxa	Three and over, although it can be used on younger kids in a well-ventilated room	Can be used over large areas Useful on points such as Ki 1 to attract heat downwards	Risk of small pieces of ash dropping; produces a lot of smoke (unless smokeless moxa is used) Not so good for small points on young kids

Direct moxa	Approximately six and upwards depending on maturity	Little smoke; effective way of tonifying	Not so good for warming areas Not appropriate for babies and toddlers May create a sudden, intense sting if left on too long
Stick-on moxa	Approximately three and over, depending on maturity	Lacks the "sting" of direct moxa; stays in place well if the child moves Gentle build-up of warmth	May be a little more time consuming than other methods
Electric moxa	Any age	No smoke	Lacks that "magic" quality of using artemisia

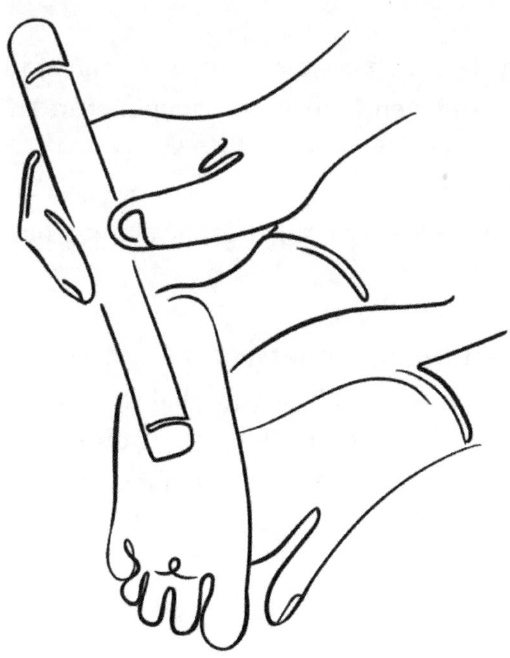

Chinese herbal medicine

What is it?

Chinese herbal medicine is the use of mainly plants, but also some minerals and animal products, to treat Chinese medicine patterns of imbalance. Herbs are most commonly taken internally in the form of granules, decoctions or tablets. At times, they can be applied to the surface of the skin too.

What age group can you use it with?

Chinese herbal medicine is most commonly used from around the age of six months upwards, when the child begins to eat foods other than just milk. However, even before this age, it can be taken by a breastfeeding mother in order to influence the child's health.

What are its main strengths?

I most commonly use Chinese herbal medicine in children in the following situations:

- In long-term, chronic conditions that are unlikely to respond sufficiently to weekly acupuncture treatments.
- In severe, complicated conditions.
- In skin conditions.
- In children who cannot get to the clinic often enough for acupuncture.

What are its main weaknesses?

The obvious weakness of Chinese herbal medicine for children is their reluctance to take it. The taste is often not appealing. Once a child is old enough to swallow tablets, this makes things easier, although tablets are arguably less effective than granules or decoctions.

Top tips when using Chinese herbal medicine

- I tend to prescribe Chinese herbs as granules in young children, and either granules, capsules or tablets in older children.

- In order to raise the chances of gaining compliance with the child, start with a very low dose of herbs. A tiny amount of herbs sprinkled in granule form over food for a period of a couple of weeks will help the child to acclimatize to the taste of the herbs.

- My feeling is that it does not really matter to what lengths we need to go to disguise the taste of the herbs, as long as the child ingests them. I draw the line at Coca-Cola!

- It tends to work better for the child to have all their herbs in one spoonful of food than to mix the herbs in an entire portion. This way they can have one mouthful they may not be too keen on and then enjoy the rest of the meal.

- If either we or the parent set up an expectation with the child that the herbs taste disgusting, the child will find the herbs disgusting. How we and the parents present the idea of the herbs to the child is therefore crucial.

A thorough training in Chinese herbal medicine is required in order to prescribe herbs to children. Practitioners must also have appropriate insurance cover. Please research the level of qualification required in your country and relevant accredited courses.

Cupping

What is it?

Cupping involves placing cups on the body to create suction. There are many different types of cupping, including Fire cupping and Water cupping. When working with children of all ages, I use silicone cups. They are well tolerated and effective. They avoid the need to use a flame.

When treating adults with cupping, the practitioner usually wants and expects to see strong red or purple markings which indicate that the treatment has created some movement in the blood and has been effective. Very few children suffer from blood stagnation, and our aims when cupping children are different. Please see the "What are its main strengths?" section for further explanation of this.

Most of the time, I use a flash-cupping technique with my silicone cups (this is why in my clinic cups are known as "the kissing machine," because the sound it makes is similar to the sound of a kiss). This is a *yang* technique and resonates with a child's *yang* energy. I may sometimes use static cups too.

What age group can you use it with?

It's possible to buy tiny silicone cups, and to buy cups of different firmness too. This makes it possible to use cups even on babies and toddlers, although, of course, on this age group, we would use tiny and very soft cups.

What are its main strengths?

Cups can be used on acupuncture points, along channels or over areas. I use cupping in children in the following situations:

- To loosen thick phlegm.
- To disperse heat.
- To move *qi*.
- To tonify deficiencies.

More specifically, I find cupping invaluable in the treatment of the following symptoms:

- On the back in lung conditions.
- Over the relevant back *shu* points to either disperse or tonify an organ.
- Over the sinuses when there is congestion or blockage.
- Over the abdomen (following the course of the intestines) to promote peristalsis in a child who is constipated.

What are its main weaknesses?

It may sound like a strange weakness, but children generally love cupping so much that they want it every time they come for a treatment. However, because it is so versatile, it is usually possible to incorporate it into your treatment, whatever it is that is presenting. Occasionally, children find cupping too ticklish, but this is rare.

Top tips when using cupping

- Choose the right size and firmness of cup to match the child. The more excess the child, or the more excess the condition, the firmer the cup.

- When you are trying to disperse or clear, use a fast, strong flash-cupping technique. When you are trying to tonify, use a slow, gentle technique.

- I sometimes recommend to the parents of children who are prone to croup and nasty chesty coughs that they buy a cup they can keep at home. I show them how and where to use it and in what situation they might use it.

- If your cupping has left any marks, it is vital that you send them away with a letter explaining what you have done.

This is so that anyone the child comes into contact with understands the child has not come to any harm.

Gua sha

What is it?

Gua sha involves strongly stroking a tool (known as a *gua sha ban*) over the surface of the skin, which has been lubricated with oil. *Gua sha bans* may be made from different materials and come in different shapes and sizes. Obviously, when working with children, small ones are more apt.

When performed on adults, *gua sha* is a strong technique which can feel quite intense for the patient and produce very strong red or purple petechiae (known as *sha*). As is the case with every method we may use when treating children, they do not require nearly such strong intervention as an adult might. Therefore, when we perform *gua sha*, we should approach it in a gentle manner and only go to a level that the child can happily tolerate. Similarly, we really do not need to elicit the same degree or intensity of *sha* that we would on an adult. A small amount of redness is normally quite sufficient to create the desired therapeutic effect.

What age group can you use it with?

Gua sha can theoretically be used on any age group. However, I only very rarely use it on babies and toddlers.

What are its main strengths?

Gua sha is useful in the following clinical situations:

- To release the exterior.
- To clear excess heat. *Gua sha* has an "opening" effect at the surface of the body, providing a pathway via which a heat pathogen can escape.

- To move *qi* and blood. I tend to only need to do this in older children who come to the clinic with sports injuries.

What are its main weaknesses?

Some children simply cannot tolerate the feeling of *gua sha*. However, this is not generally problematic, as there are always other methods we can use to achieve the desired therapeutic effect.

There are also a small proportion of children who may worry about the marks that *gua sha* leave. With pre-teens and teenagers, it is important to check with them before you do *gua sha* that they are happy for there to be some discoloration for some time afterwards.

Top tips when using gua sha

- I tend to use a neutral oil, such as olive or grapeseed oil, rather than the strong, pungent oils often used with adults. I find that children often can't tolerate the smell of the pungent oils, and they are too heating for many children anyway. Be sure to check with the parent about possible allergies before you apply any oil.

- Support the part of the body upon which you are doing the *gua sha*. This makes it more comfortable for the child. So if, for example, you are doing it on the back, have one hand on the top of the child's shoulder.

- Hold the *gua sha ban* at an oblique angle, rather than at a 90-degree angle to the skin. This will mitigate against any "sharp" feeling.

- Hold the *gua sha ban* so that the backs of your fingers touch the skin, along with the *gua sha ban*. This dilutes the intensity of the feeling, making it easier for a child to tolerate.

- Always make sure that you send any child who has had *gua sha* home with a letter explaining what you have done. This is so that anyone the child comes into contact with understands the child has not come to any harm.

Summary

Most of us tend to have certain treatment modalities with which we resonate and feel more comfortable. However, the more we can expand our range of "tools" with which we can treat children, the more children we will be able to help. The traditional methods described in this chapter can be used to treat a wide range of different aged children of different personality types, as well as a wide range of pathologies. However, they may not be enough to successfully treat every child. In the next chapter, we will look at modern treatment methods, the existence of which has expanded the possibilities of treating children.

CHAPTER 8

Modern Methods of Treating Children

When I first became an acupuncturist, I considered myself a traditionalist. My natural inclination was that the traditional ways were the best ways. As I started to see more and more children, I was forced to become more open-minded. Now, 25 years on, I would describe myself as a huge fan of modern innovations. This is because I have come to realize that these innovations mean we can help far more children than we would otherwise.

To some degree, as I have adopted these modern treatment modalities, I have had to work them out as I have gone along. There is very little about most of them in the literature. I have also benefitted hugely from discussions with colleagues who treat children. What I present below is based largely on the lessons I have learned, and the mistakes I have made, from my clinical experience. I urge readers to take this as a guide but also to adapt my suggestions in a way that fits the needs of each particular situation.

It is beyond the scope of this book to teach all the methods described in this chapter from scratch. This chapter is intended to make practitioners aware of the many treatment modalities there are available. I have indicated throughout when the reader needs to access further training or resources. Please see the "Further resources" section for more information on this.

Electrical treatment methods

Laser acupuncture

What is it?

Laser acupuncture involves stimulating acupuncture points with the use of therapeutic light. This is done with a laser pen, which is held over one acupuncture point for a specified period of time. It is possible to buy a laser pen which emits any of the following types of light:

- Red light
- Infrared light
- Blue light.

As well as laser pens, there are many other laser devices on the market. I do not have experience of using these, and they are out of reach financially for most practitioners, which is why I limit my discussion below to the use of laser pens.

What age group can you use it with?

Laser acupuncture can be used with any age group, all the way from newborns to teenagers.

What are its main strengths?

Laser acupuncture is an amazing innovation for pediatrics because it is entirely painless. In my opinion, a good laser pen enables us to get as close as possible to the effect we can get with a needle. This has really been a game changer for the pediatric practitioner. With a laser pen, it is possible to treat almost any point on the body and for the child to barely even know they are receiving a treatment. I often combine laser and needles in the same treatment. For example, there are some children who are happy to be needled on their limbs but not on their backs, where we can use a laser in lieu of a needle.

Depending on the capacity of the practitioner's laser pen, it is often possible to set it to emit a particular dose of light at any one point and also to change the rate at which the light is emitted as well as the particular resonance of the light. This means that we can adapt how we use a laser pen specifically to meet the needs of the individual child.

What are its main weaknesses?

In my experience, laser pens are not effective when treating *yin* pathogens such as damp or phlegm. There are also some important cautions and contraindications of which we should be aware before using laser acupuncture:

- Do not use it near the eye. Although it's possible for the child to wear protective glasses, I tend to avoid eye points altogether when using laser.
- Do not use it on open fontanelles on a baby.
- Do not use it on the testicles.
- Do not use it on cancerous or pre-cancerous tumors.
- Do not use it on skin which is damaged due to UV light or radiation.
- Do not use it on the head in a child with epilepsy.

Top tips when using laser acupuncture

- Hold the laser pen perpendicular so that none of the therapeutic light "escapes" when you are treating a point.

- If you have a laser pen which beeps when the treatment is

done, ask the child to listen out for and count the beeps as a way of engaging them with the treatment.

- Keep a firm hand on your laser pen at all times. Anything with buttons is usually appealing to a child, and it is not safe for them to have it in their hands (nor is it safe for the laser pen!).

- If you have a laser pen with different settings, be sure to write in your notes which setting you use at each treatment so you know for the next time.

- Wipe the tip of the laser with an alcohol wipe between each treatment.

Choosing the right laser pen

When it comes to buying a laser pen, it is true that you get what you pay for. There are some laser pens on the market which cost a few hundred dollars, but their effectiveness is limited. There are others which cost somewhere between $2000 and $6000 which are very effective.

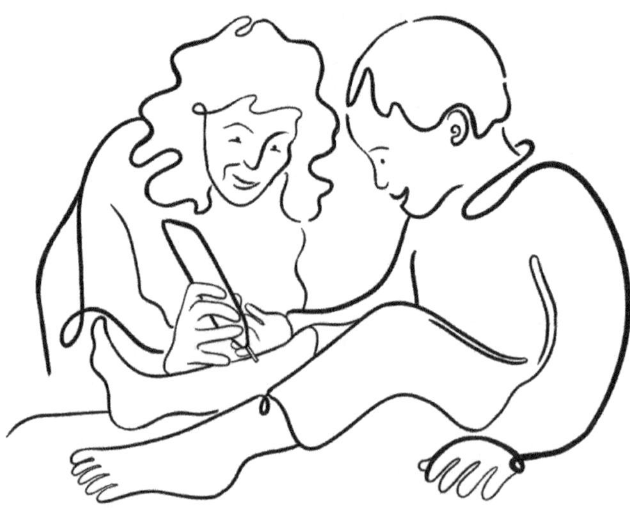

One of the most important decisions to make before buying a laser pen is which kind of laser light you want it to emit. Red or infrared light is mostly used for tonifying, although at low frequencies it can be used for dispersing. Blue laser light is only really effective for dispersing, pain relief and the treatment of acute conditions.

I highly advise finding either an in-person or online course before introducing laser into your practice, in order to make sure you know how to use it safely. It is also wise to check whether your insurance covers you for using laser.

Cutaneous electrical stimulation (CES)

What is it?

Cutaneous electrical stimulation (CES) is the use of electric current to stimulate an acupuncture point directly on the skin instead of via a needle. There are two possible ways of doing this:

- By using a probe (which comes with an electro-acupuncture machine) and holding it directly on the skin at an acupuncture point.
- By placing damp cotton balls in crocodile clips and placing them on the skin, on two different acupuncture points which are close together.* The damp cotton balls both help to increase comfort and conduct electricity.

What age group can you use it with?

In order to safely and comfortably use CES, the child must be able to give us feedback about what they are feeling. They need also to be trusted not to interfere with the controls on the electro-device.

* I learned this method of using CES from the late and very great Alex Tiberi.

For these two reasons, I tend to use it on children from around six or seven years old and upwards, depending on their maturity.

What are its main strengths?

CES is a great alternative to needles when we want to either tonify or sedate. It can be used on any acupuncture point on the body but is especially useful on points where children are less likely to tolerate needles, such as points on the face. Here are some specific clinical situations where I find CES especially useful:

- On all the points surrounding the eye for almost any eye complaint, including strabismus, myopia, conjunctivitis.
- On points near the nose, such as LI 20 and *bitong*, in chronic conditions affecting the nose, such as hay fever.
- On points around the ear (e.g., SJ 17, SJ 22, SI 19, GB 2) for glue ear or hearing loss.
- On points around the jaw (e.g., SI 17) for teeth grinding.
- On the sacral points in a child who is bedwetting.
- On hard or swollen lymph nodes (usually indicative of a Lingering Pathogen Factor) in order to encourage them to dissipate.

What are its main weaknesses?

Many children tolerate CES very well and actually enjoy "the tickle machine."* Others, however, really do not enjoy it. They find the sensation, even at its weakest, too intense, and there is something about the quality of it that makes them feel agitated. To some degree, you never know how a particular child will find it until you try. On the other hand, I find that deficient, sensitive and nervous children are least likely to enjoy it.

* My friend and colleague in California, David Allen, coined this term "the tickle machine."

Top tips when using CES

- CES will not work unless you have an electro-machine with a relatively high output. This is because you are using it without needles.
- It is essential to place the damp cotton balls or probe, whichever you are using, on the skin when the electro-device is turned down to zero. I then ask the child to very slowly turn the dial up until they begin to feel a tingle. They can then increase it if they feel they can manage it. Children like having control of the buttons! This also frees you up to be managing the probe or crocodile clips.
- I find that CES is most effective when you have your electro-device on a slow, pulsating frequency.

Table 8.1 shows how to differentiate between tonifying and dispersing with CES.

Table 8.1 Differentiating between tonifying and dispersing with CES

Tonifying	Dispersing
Short period of time (up to 20 seconds)	Longer period of time (30–60 seconds)
Lower frequency (below 5 Hz)	Higher frequency (above 5 Hz)
Lower intensity	Higher intensity

If you are not familiar with using an electro-device in this way, I highly recommend that you try it out on yourself or a family member. Build up your confidence in this way before introducing it with children in your clinic.

Microcurrent stimulation

What is it?

Microcurrent stimulation is performed using a small, pen-sized machine. The tip of the machine is held over an acupuncture point which passes a barely feelable microcurrent through it. Depending on the machine, it usually needs to be held in place for between 5 and 20 seconds. There are many different microcurrent machines on the market, and I encourage readers to do some research, chat to colleagues and find one that suits their budget.

What age group can you use it with?

Microcurrent stimulation can be used with any age group. When using it on body points, I tend to use it on children up to the age of about six. In older children, I find it is not quite powerful enough, unless combined with another treatment method.

What are its main strengths?

Microcurrent stimulation is especially useful in the following situations:

- When doing auricular therapy—it's a painless way of stimulating ear points and can also be used to locate them accurately too.
- When we want to stimulate a body point on a young child who will not tolerate needles, in the absence of a laser pen.

What are its main weaknesses?

Microcurrent stimulation is great up to a certain point, but ultimately remains a low dose treatment so is limited in its capacity.

Top tip when using microcurrent stimulation

- Most microcurrent pens have a point finder function too. This is useful on very little ears where there are a lot of points in a very small area!

Treatment using stickers

The following treatment modalities all involve stickers, i.e., sticking something on to the skin at an acupuncture point in order to stimulate it. There are some general guidelines to bear in mind when using any kind of stick-on point stimulation, which I outline now before discussing the different types.

- Send the parent and child home with clear, written instructions about when to take the stickers off.

- Children sometimes feel agitated by the feeling of a sticker when we first apply it. The vast majority of the time, however, they will forget it is there after a minute or two. So it's helpful to support them through that first minute or two by encouraging their focus away from the sticker or simply being alongside them as they get used to the feeling.

- When children have a fear of having stickers, it is most commonly related to how it will feel to have the sticker taken off! I often advise families to take them off in the bath or to put a little bit of oil around the sticker, which will help it to peel off more easily. Some children also prefer to take the stickers off themselves so they remain in control.

- It is a mistake to think, "The longer I leave any kind of point stimulation on, the more impact it will have." There is no magic amount of time that it's possible to say is the right amount of time for each child. The key is to find the range within which our treatment is effective. This comes with experience.

I believe it is important to decide on and specify when a sticker should be removed. This is partly how we set intention. To some degree, this is dictated by practicalities. For example, I may put stickers on at the end of a treatment I give the child in the late afternoon and ask them to take them off either just before they go to bed (in a younger child) or the following morning before school (in an older child). I may ask that the stickers are left on overnight if their purpose is to ease a symptom that flares during the night, for example, a phlegmy cough.

In my opinion, it is never a good policy to leave a point being stimulated day after day. Therefore, when necessary, I give parents extra stickers to take home and ask them to take a photograph and mark the point when they remove a sticker. If they are coming off in the morning, for example, I may then ask them to put a new sticker on that evening. Table 8.2 outlines the main considerations when deciding how long stickers should be left on a point.

Table 8.2 Factors influencing sticker retention time

Shorter retention time	Longer retention time
Babies, toddlers and children under the age of eight	Children above the age of eight and teenagers
Tonification	Dispersion or sedation
Sensitive or "xu" child	Robust or "shi" child

We will now look at the different kinds of stickers that can be used to stimulate acupuncture points.

Press spheres, seeds or balls

What are they?

Press spheres, seeds or tiny balls are sold attached to the middle of a small, round, hypoallergenic sticker. They are placed directly on the skin, on either body or ear points. There are many different varieties available, and I encourage practitioners to find what is available in their country and experiment to see which they find the easiest to work with and most effective.

What age group can you use them with?

Press spheres, seeds and balls can be used on any age group but, because they are low dose, they tend to be used most commonly on babies and young children.

What are their main strengths?

Press spheres, seeds or balls can be chosen depending on the therapeutic effect we want to achieve. For example:

- Gold spheres can be used on points we want to tonify.
- Silver spheres can be used on points we want to disperse.
- Mustard seeds can be used on points we want to warm.

What are their main weaknesses?

Press spheres, seeds or balls are low dose so are of limited value in older children and teens. In babies and toddlers who are in the oral phase, great care must be taken that they are not placed anywhere that the child could peel them off and put them in their mouth. Occasionally, the tape which is used to stick them to the skin may cause irritation.

Top tips when using press spheres, seeds and balls

- Place a little piece of micropore tape over the sticker to prevent it falling off.
- Ask parents to check in with the seeds every night to make sure the skin is not reacting.

Magnet therapy

My understanding and use of magnets has been hugely informed by my fellow practitioner Jong Baik* to whom I would like to give great thanks.

What is it?

Magnet therapy involves the use of magnets as a way of stimulating acupuncture points. Even though magnet therapy in

* www.jongbaik.co.uk

TEAMs has a long history,* I include it in this chapter on modern methods because the way we use them today has been shaped by modern technical innovations.

Magnets are made from highly polished hematite and may be coated in nickel. Only magnets with a clearly labelled "north" and "south" side should be used. When using single magnets, the "north" side of the magnet should be applied to the skin, never the south side. Magnets are usually applied during a treatment session with a sticker, and instructions are given to the parents about when to take them off. One magnet may be applied to a specific acupuncture point or an *ahshi* point. Several magnets may be applied to a wider area of pain or disease (again, always with the north side of the magnet applied to the skin).

What age group can you use it with?

Magnets can be used on all children providing the cautions and contraindications below are followed.

What strength of magnet should I use?

Magnet strength is measured in gauss. Whilst there is no definite guide as to what strength magnet should be used at which age, Table 8.3 indicates the strength I use based on what I have been taught and my research into it and what I find works in the clinic.

Table 8.3 Determining magnet strength

Low strength magnets (around 100–200 gauss)	Higher strength magnets (between 200–800 guass)
Babies, toddlers and children under the age of eight	Children above the age of eight and teenagers
Chronic conditions	Acute conditions
Sensitive or "xu" child	Robust or "shi" child

* Magnet therapy is mentioned in the *Shen Nong Ben Cao Jing* and the *Beiji Qian Jin Yao Fang*, for example.

How long should a magnet be left on a point?

There are several factors which determine how long a magnet should be left on a point. As with choosing the strength, there is no definite guide, but there are helpful guidelines, which I have outlined in Table 8.3. In my opinion, it is wrong to think that the longer a magnet is left on, the better. Dosage is everything, and we need to find the "therapeutic window" for each child. As a general rule of thumb, I ask children to leave their magnets on for anywhere between six hours and three days. Any longer than this, and I believe that the acupuncture point stops reacting to the magnet, and the overall therapeutic effect is reduced.

Cautions and contraindications

Magnets should not be applied in any of the following situations:

- On a young child in the oral phase to a part of the body where they could potentially peel the magnet off and put it in their mouth.
- On a child with a pacemaker or a hearing aid (magnets may interfere with their functioning).
- Near the heart.
- If symptoms such as yawning, dizziness or tingling occur.
- Magnets should be removed if skin irritation occurs.

What are its main strengths?

Magnet therapy's greatest strengths are that it is entirely painless and that it enables a child to continue receiving a low dose of treatment after their session and between sessions. When using magnets, we are able to differentiate whether we want to tonify or disperse depending on the color of magnet we use (silver-coated magnets are dispersing and gold-coated ones are tonifying). As there are different strengths of magnets on the market, we are able to tailor our treatment to suit the age and constitution of the child.

As well as being used as an alternative to a needle on an acupuncture point, magnets may also be used for the following symptoms:

- Swelling
- Pain
- Local inflammation.

Another strength of magnet therapy is that it may be used when we want to ameliorate a specific symptom to which the child is prone, such as a cough or asthma. We can give the parents magnets, illustrations and instructions so that when the symptom arises, they can apply a magnet with the aim of lessening the severity of the symptom.

What are its main weaknesses?

In my experience, magnets take a little time to have a therapeutic effect. When treating acute conditions, the effect is unlikely to be as immediate as it would be when using a needle, for example.

Press needles

What are they?

Press needles, sometimes known as press tacks, are micro acupuncture needles which can be left in situ on acupuncture points for a period of time. There are various different types of press needles including apex needles and intradermal needles. My experience of press needles is solely with Pyonex needles, which are extremely small and have the same sharpness as the best quality filiform needles.

What age group can you use them with?

Pyonex press needles come in different sizes, and the smallest ones can be used even on babies. However, I most commonly use press needles on children from the age of approximately four or five upwards. The reason for this is that younger children simply do not need this level of treatment dose. Seeds or small magnets are usually sufficient to bring about the desired effects.

What are their main strengths?

Press needles are extremely effective in the following situations:

- To use on children who will not tolerate regular acupuncture needles.
- To disperse a pathogen such as heat or damp, and to move *qi*.
- When we want to continue the treatment we have done in clinic after the child leaves.

What are their main weaknesses?

My experience is that press needles are far more effective at dispersing than they are tonifying. However, I have colleagues who use press needles whether or not they are dispersing or tonifying. As with everything, I urge readers to try one approach and see both how it feels to them and what results they get. There is no one approach to how we treat. The most important thing is always to be clear about what you are doing and why you are doing it, and to have consistency.

The reason I believe press needles are not as effective for tonifying is because when a needle is left in situ for as long as press needles usually are (i.e., for several hours or even a few days), the *qi* inevitably becomes more and more dispersed.

To tonify or disperse, that is the question!

When I teach practitioners who all have very different trainings and use different styles of acupuncture, one of the things I find that varies most is their opinions on tonification and dispersion. On one end of the spectrum, there are those who believe it is vital that you are clear before you insert a needle whether you want to tonify or disperse and that you change your needle technique accordingly. On the other end of the spectrum are those who believe that this does not really matter because the body will respond to the needle however it needs to.

I am firmly in the former camp. Medicine is intention, and the clearer our intention, the more effective our treatments. It is especially important when we are leaving anything in situ, whether it be a press needle, seed or magnet, to be clear about whether our intention is to tonify or disperse.

Top tips when using press needles

- If using Pyonex, start with the smallest size you think will be effective. If necessary, work your way up. If you initially put on too big a size and the child finds it uncomfortable, they may never let you put another on again!

- Be safe! Although they are tiny, press needles are still needles. Check with your professional body about their rules for using retained needles. Think through potential hazards—for example, young siblings peeling them off and putting them in their mouths. I only ever send kids home with press needles if I think they and their parents can manage them safely. I also never send a child home with a press needle who will be going to school or daycare after the treatment.

- Give parents a mini sharps box or suggest they have a small jam jar in which to dispose of the press needles. They can then bring them back to you at the next appointment, and you can dispose of them safely.

Essential oil acutherapy

My understanding and use of essential oils has been highly informed by several teachers, namely Peter Holmes, Tiffany Carole and Jeffrey Yuen, to all of whom I am extremely grateful.

What is it?

Essential oil acutherapy (EOA) is the use of essential oils on acupuncture points or via inhalation according to their Chinese medicine properties.* Although aromatic substances have been used in Asian culture for all of recorded history, there is no known use of essential oils within TEAMs until the very late 20th century, when essential oil production was first developed.[41] Essential oils gain their efficacy from the fact that they embody the *jing* of a plant. Therefore, when we introduce them to the body via the acupuncture channel system, they are able to modulate the *jing, qi,* and *shen* of the body.

Essential oils can be applied to acupuncture points instead of needles. Alternatively, we may choose oils to address the root *ben* of a problem and needles to address the *biao,* or vice versa. We could apply oils to certain distal acupuncture points while needling other proximal points, for example. We can use oils in the clinic or instruct families how to use them at home. The possibilities are limitless!

What age group can you use it with?

EOA can be used with any age group from six months and above. It is essential to dilute the essential oil on younger age groups.

What are its main strengths?

EOA is a totally painless way of bringing back balance to the body. Children tend to resonate with it and enjoy smelling the oils. It's a gentle yet powerful way to access *qi* in the acupuncture

---

* Essential oils can also be taken internally, but I do not use this method with children and therefore do not cover it here.

channels and can be used in both acute and chronic conditions. There are essential oils for every pattern of imbalance that we may come across. I find children highly responsive to essential oils, and it is one of my most favored treatment modalities.

What are its main weaknesses?

There are really no weaknesses in terms of what EOA can do for the patient. A minor drawback is that some children are hypersensitive to any kind of smell and may not tolerate it, but this is unusual. I find that most of the time children are drawn towards the smell of an oil that energetically fits their imbalance.

Cautions and contraindications

The vast majority of the time, essential oils can be used with extremely good results and without any negative reactions. However, they are potent and powerful so should always be used mindfully and with a thorough knowledge and understanding of the properties of each oil. This is why I strongly recommend practitioners interested in incorporating them into their practice undertake a thorough training. They key cautions and contraindications to be aware of are as follows:

- Skin irritation may occur with even tiny amounts of any diluted oils on some children; therefore, it is essential to go slowly and use a tiny amount of diluted oil on one point and wait before proceeding any further.

- Certain oils are known to sensitize the skin and may cause allergic reactions.

- Certain oils are known to increase the skin's sensitivity when exposed to sunlight.

- Poor essential oil quality may increase the incidence of an adverse reaction.

Top tips when using EOA

- If there is more than one oil that fits with the pattern of imbalance you want to treat, ask the child to smell two oils and choose the one they are most drawn to. I advise against asking them to choose between more than two, as this can be too much choice for a little person.

- If you are asking parents to apply essential oil at home, send them home with written instructions which stress how little they need to use on each point. Less really is more when it comes to essential oils.

- When starting out using essential oils in your clinic, I would advise investing in just a small number of oils. As a practitioner, it's important that you slowly build up a relationship with an oil over time. You can gradually increase the number of oils you hold in your clinic over time.

- Having tried many methods, I now use a toothpick to apply essential oil to acupuncture points. Cotton earbuds absorb too much of the oil, which is wasteful. Almost everything else is too big and means you end up using too much oil on each point.

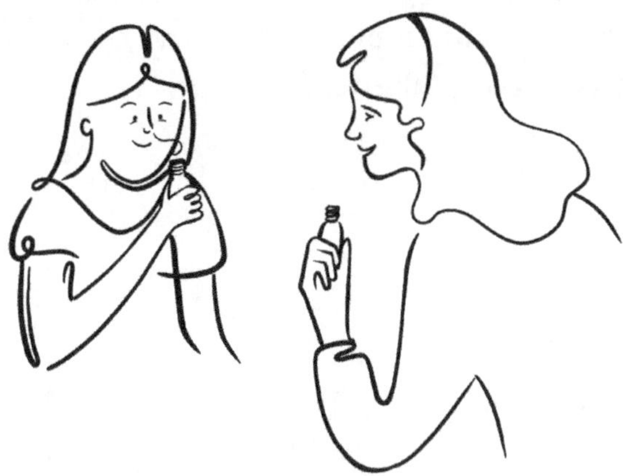

I highly recommend learning about the Chinese medicine energetics of essential oils from several excellent books on the subject or from one of several TEAMs practitioners who lecture on this subject (please see the "Further resources" section).

Summary

The modalities described in this chapter are the ones I use every day, alongside the traditional methods described in the previous chapter. I encourage readers to try out as many different ways of delivering their treatment as possible but also to avoid being, "a jack of all trades and a master of none." Rather than endeavoring to incorporate many new modalities at the same time, I would suggest picking one which most appeals to you and honing the skill of using it before going on to learn another modality.

Different modalities resonate with different practitioners. You may find you immediately "click" with some of them, and others may feel awkward for you. You can probably use your favored modalities most of the time, but there may be occasions when the particular proclivities of a particular child mean you need to turn to a modality you are not quite so at ease with. It is my believe that if we have a good diagnosis and think that TEAMs can help a child, the onus is on us to find a way of delivering their treatment that is acceptable to them.

CHAPTER 9

How to Choose and Combine Treatment Modalities

When I first studied pediatrics, I remember my teacher and friend Julian Scott saying to me, "The difficulty of treating children is finding a way to deliver their treatment." At the time, I did not fully appreciate just how apt that statement was. Over the years of treating children, I have come to understand that Julian had hit the nail right on the head. A significant number of children who come to see us will not be happy to accept being needled, certainly not at first and often not in the places or to the degree that we feel they need. Therefore, if we want to treat children successfully, we need to be flexible and creative in how we go about delivering treatment.

As outlined in Chapters 7 and 8, thankfully we have so many different modalities available with which to treat children. Whilst this chapter explores how to go about choosing the right modalities for each child and how to combine them, I would like to stress here that there is no "one way." There may be "wrong ways," but there is more than one "right way." As always, we must respond in the moment to the child in front of us. As you get to know a child, you will understand what approach will work for them.

Choosing and combining treatment modalities

There can be an inherent tension when treating children between what we want to do in terms of treatment and what the child will accept. This can be difficult. We may see a child who is struggling with a particular symptom, and we may know that if we could do a particular treatment, we would have a good chance of helping it. However, it is a pyrrhic victory to force a treatment on a child who does not want it. It harms our therapeutic relationship with them and may mean they never want to have acupuncture again. Playing the long game is usually the best policy. Deepening our rapport with a child and allowing their trust in us to grow optimizes the chances of us moving towards doing the treatment we know will best help them. In the meantime, we can call upon some of the many treatment modalities available to us. The ones the child will accept may not be our first choice but are "good enough" to begin helping the child whilst protecting our long-term therapeutic relationship.

It is also important to stress that how we approach treatment is not fixed. It is an ever-changing entity. A treatment modality that is not acceptable to a child initially may be welcomed further along in the treatment journey. Conversely, a child may be happy to have needles for months but then something changes. They have a hospital visit which creates a needle phobia or they simply go through a different stage of development. Every single time we see a child, we need to reassess and check if they are happy with what we propose before we begin treatment.

Here are some questions to ask yourself when deciding which treatment modalities to use with a particular child:

- Which are the optimum treatment modalities to use to treat this child and their condition?
- Is the child open to these modalities?

- If not, what is my next best modality to use in order to help the child?
- What is the block for this child in receiving a particular modality (e.g., unfamiliarity, lack of understanding, fear of pain)?
- Is there anything I can do to help the child to get past the block (e.g., demonstrating on myself or the parent, explaining the process)?
- How do the potential gains of pushing a certain treatment modality compare with the potential losses?
- Are there certain treatment modalities that the child is not yet open to but I can work towards using in the future?

Below I outline some cases in order to illustrate how we might go about combining different treatment modalities.

Holly—nine-year-old with bedwetting

Modalities used in clinic: *shonishin*, moxibustion, laser therapy, magnet therapy

Modalities used at home: pediatric *tui na*

Holly was very clear from the start that she did not want to be needled. I took this seriously, as she looked petrified when I showed her my tiny needles and demonstrated on her mum!

Diagnosis

Earth constitutional imbalance; Spleen and Kidney *yang* deficiency; back family circulation phase*; scar interference (Holly

* This diagnosis is based on Dr. Thomas Wernicke's *shonishin* style. Please see *Shonishin: The Art of Non-Invasive Acupuncture* for further details.

had had a large birth mark removed at one year old, which covered the Bladder channel on her right calf).

A typical treatment

- Back family *shonishin* treatment.
- *Shonishin* over the scar.
- Electric moxa on points such as Bl 23 *shenshu* and Bl 28 *pangguangshu.*
- Laser pen on a variety of Spleen, Kidney and Bladder points (perhaps two or three per treatment).

Home treatment

- Sent home with magnets on two Spleen or Kidney points.
- Taught Mum a *tui na* routine to support the Spleen and Kidneys to perform every evening.

Rationale

I believed that Holly's imbalances stemmed from the surgery across her Bladder channel at one year old and her response (based on her Earth constitution) to a difficult time in her family around the ages of three to five years old. *Shonishin* is the best way I know to treat scar interference and also to treat problems which arise due to a developmental imbalance.

Whenever there is *yang* deficiency, some sort of moxa is an obvious choice. In Holly's case, I chose electric moxa because I felt she was too nervous to have direct moxa. I could equally have chosen pole moxa or stick-on moxa.

I used a laser pen to tonify the Spleen and Kidneys as, in my experience, red or infrared laser light is the next best way to tonify if you cannot use needles.

Bedwetting can need a lot of treatment before seeing a positive response. This is why I chose to back up what I was doing in clinic with magnets and with Holly's mum doing some pediatric *tui na* at home. I would have liked to prescribe herbs, but Holly was a very fussy eater, could not swallow tablets and was not open to this.

Progression

Holly remained adamant that she did not want to try needles, or even Pyonex stickers. However, she did allow me to try some stick-on moxa and preferred that to electric moxa. Holly is a good example of a sensitive child who responded well to relatively low-dose treatments. Even at the age of nine, we were able to get a good treatment outcome without using needles.

Leo—four-year-old with food allergies

Modalities used in clinic: pediatric *tui na*; press needles; cupping; laser acupuncture

Diagnosis: Food Accumulation; Liver heat; Spleen *qi* deficiency

A typical treatment

- Pediatric *tui na* to move Food Accumulation, clear Liver heat and disperse the Liver and tonify the Spleen.
- Flash cupping around the hypochondrial area and abdomen to move Food Accumulation.
- Press needles on points to disperse the Liver.
- Laser therapy on points to tonify the Spleen.

Rationale

Leo was young enough to use pediatric *tui na* as the mainstay of his treatment. In his age group, even entirely on its own, it is very effective. Pediatric *tui na* relaxed Leo, and there are moves to address each of his three key pathologies. Flash cupping is a powerful way of moving *qi* locally, and Leo absolutely loved it. So I used it at every treatment around the hypochondrium and abdomen, both of which felt distended and warm.

I noticed when I first used press needles (on points such as Liv 3 *taichong* and Liv 2 *xingjiang*) that Leo was very sensitive to them. I had to use the smallest size otherwise he would hate the feeling and I would have to take it off. This is what made me think he was not ready to try needles. Press needles are a great way to move and disperse *qi* or pathogens, so it did not matter. Laser acupuncture (AKA "the beepy machine") is a strong way to tonify so I would usually finish off Leo's treatment by choosing a couple of points that strengthened and supported the Spleen.

Progression

Leo is now seven and still comes for treatments once a month to maintain the progress we made. When he first came, his mum encouraged him to try a needle. He was adamant he would not do this, and I explained I could treat him successfully without using needles. Occasionally, I gently asked if he wanted to try one, but the answer was always a very clear "no."

However, a few months ago, Leo turned up for his treatment and said his classmate told him he had needles when he came to see me and he wanted them too. He was almost cross, as if he were missing out! So, now I use needles on Leo instead of Pyonex and laser. Sometimes, it is not what we do but something outside of our control that changes a child's mind about needles.

Rosalind—11-year-old with attention deficit hyperactivity disorder (ADHD)

Modalities used in clinic: needles, then pediatric *tui na* and channel massages and laser acupuncture, then needles again!

Modalities used at home: herbs

Diagnosis: Heart and Liver blood deficiency; phlegm misting the Mind; heat agitating the *shen*

A typical treatment

- Needles, usually on about five or six points per session, to address Rosalind's patterns of imbalance.

- After about six months of treatment, Rosalind went through a phase of resistance when she didn't want needles. At this point, I switched to some pediatric *tui na*, as well as channel massages and laser. In this age group, I find the pediatric *tui na* moves on the head and torso are still effective. After three or four sessions, I gradually introduced needles again, and Rosalind has been fine with them ever since. Her phase of not wanting needles coincided with her transition to secondary school.

Home treatment

- Rosalind took Chinese herbal medicine in the form of granules at home, twice daily.

Rationale

From the start, Rosalind was entirely comfortable with needles and would obviously relax deeply whilst they were in. She loved her treatments and benefitted from them hugely. It was therefore important that, during a phase of stress in her life when she became resistant to needles, I was flexible and did not turn having them or not into a battle. I did not want her to turn away from acupuncture, a source of great support for her. When I felt that Rosalind was feeling less anxious, I very slowly suggested we try reintroducing needles, literally one needle at a time.

In hindsight, I feel that part of this phase was Rosalind feeling that some aspects of her external environment were out of control. In saying she didn't want needles, she was asserting some control in a safe environment where she felt she could do this.

I prescribed Rosalind herbs for two reasons. First, she had

three very different patterns of imbalance. Giving her herbs to nourish blood meant I was freed up in the appointments to focus my acupuncture on resolving phlegm, clearing heat and calming the *shen*. Second, Rosalind's diet was poor, so giving her blood-nourishing herbs (at the same time as dietary suggestions) seemed like a more efficient way of treating this pathology.

Progression

Rosalind continued to take herbs for about a year, and we eventually reduced her appointments to six weekly so I could check the formula she was on was still the right one and support her through adolescent changes. She came more frequently again for a few months when her periods started so I could support her blood and help to regulate her cycle. She also comes more frequently when she has exams or during times of stress, but otherwise, she comes just occasionally for maintenance treatments.

Saanvi—two-year-old with insomnia

Modalities used in clinic: needles; *gua sha*

Diagnosis: fetal toxins leading to full heat in the Liver, Heart and Stomach

A typical treatment

- Non-retained needles on approximately three points.
- *Gua sha.*

Rationale

Saanvi was one of the hottest children I have ever seen. Both she and her poor mother were exhausted, although Saanvi's exhaustion showed itself in an extreme hyperactivity and wired state. She was constantly on the move, day and night. She was too restless and fidgety to be able to stay still for any length of time. I therefore decided that the most effective treatment for Saanvi was simply to needle her, and on this age group it's not necessary to retain the needles at all.

By just using non-retained needles, it meant the treatment could be over in a few seconds, which suited Saanvi very well. I did some gentle *gua sha* to open up the surface of the body to provide an "escape route" for the heat. This needed to be done "on the move"!

I didn't give Saanvi's mum anything to do at home. She was too exhausted to be able to take anything on and, as a single parent, it would have been very hard for her to carry out any pediatric *tui na* on her own.

Progression

As often happens when we are clearing fetal toxins, after four treatments, Saanvi had a big fever. I communicated with her mum during the fever to help her support Saanvi through it. This was a big turning point and an opportunity for her to vent a huge amount of heat. Saanvi began sleeping well, although sadly her mother did not. She had almost lost the habit of sleeping. I referred Saanvi's mum to a colleague of mine who treats adults and, the last I heard, both Saanvi and her mum were doing very well.

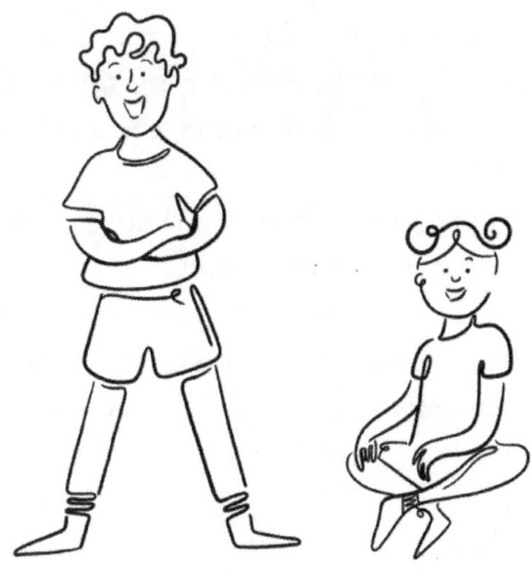

Mia—eight-year-old with anxiety

Modalities used in clinic: *shonishin*, moxibustion

Modalities used at home: essential oil therapy; magnet therapy

Diagnosis: front family circulation phase; Kidney and Heart *yin* deficiency; *shen* agitation

A typical treatment

- Front family *shonishin* treatment.
- Direct moxibustion.

Home treatment

- Application of two different essential oils in dilution on Ht 7 *shenmen* and Ki 25 *shencang*, daily.
- Essential oil inhaler tube to be used at moments of heightened anxiety.

Rationale

Mia was in a constantly hypervigilant state when she first came to see me. I started with an appropriate *shonishin* treatment and, as is often the case with *shonishin*, she would immediately become more relaxed.

I find using a small number of direct moxa cones on relevant points is an effective way of nourishing *yin* (remembering that moxa is not always warming). Mia also found this extremely relaxing and often commented that she loved the smell of the moxa smoke. This indicated to me that Mia had a strong olfactory sense and led me to think that essential oil therapy would therefore be a good modality to include in her treatment. Mia really enjoyed choosing between the two different oils that I offered her and, with her mother's guidance, diligently used them at home. She also loved keeping her "smelly tube" in her pocket at home to call upon when her anxiety began to rise.

Progression

After three months of treatment, Mia asked if she could try a needle. She felt very proud of herself when she did. When she comes to see me now, one of the first things she will tell me is whether or not today is a "needle day" or a "no-needle day." If she is feeling overstimulated, then it is more likely to be a "no-needle day." I feel it's so important for children to have this level of choice. Knowing Mia as I do, if she felt any pressure when she came for treatment, I do not believe she would come at all.

Freddie—eight-year-old with headaches and eczema

Modalities used in clinic: needles; CES

Modalities used at home: moxa

Diagnosis: Lingering Pathogenic Factor (LPF); Kidney *yang* deficiency

A typical treatment:

- Needles on points to soften phlegm.
- CES on a hard, swollen lymph node on Freddie's neck.
- Needles on point to tonify the Kidneys.

Rationale

I believed that Freddie's LPF, evidenced by his hard, swollen lymph node, was blocking the flow of "good blood" to the surface of the body, leading to his dry, cracked eczema. Using CES at each treatment on and around the lymph node is the most effective way I know of breaking up thick phlegm so the body can then expel it or transform it.

Freddie's headaches were caused by *yang* rising from the

underlying Kidney deficiency. I used needles on a variety of points to strengthen and warm Kidney *yang*. I also gave Freddie's mum a moxa pole with instructions to use it on Ki 1 *yongquan* at home. I asked her to use it twice a week and, additionally, whenever Freddie felt he thought he might feel a headache coming on. Using heat on Ki 1 *yongquan* is an effective way to draw floating *yang* downwards to the lower part of the body.

Progression

Once the lymph node on Freddie's neck had dissipated (a sign that we had resolved the LPF), we continued treatment for a short time to continue strengthening and supplementing the underlying deficiency. Freddie no longer comes for treatment. However, at our last session, I suggested to his mum that it would be a good idea to check in with how he is doing as he shows the first signs of pubertal change, knowing how much this time can tax the Kidney *qi*.

Adeba—16-year-old with severe depression

Modalities used in clinic: press needles, *tui na*

Diagnosis: Liver *qi* stagnation leading to heat

A typical treatment

- Press needles on several Liver and Gallbladder points; *tui na* moves on the head.

Rationale

It is easy to assume that a 16-year-old teenager would usually tolerate needles. However, when working with young people, making any kind of assumptions is usually unhelpful. Adeba had a history of severe trauma and was in an extremely fragile place when I first met him. The fact that he had agreed to come to the clinic was, in itself, a major step for him.

It was not until my third session with Adeba that he allowed me to do any kind of treatment. Prior to that, he just wanted to talk, and I listened to him carefully and actively to make sure that he felt safe. I showed him some press needles and he agreed to try them. After I had put the press needles in place, I did some *tui na* moves on Adeba's head, which I find very useful, even in teenagers, to calm the *shen* and the mind. Adeba had a purely excess condition, so it was not appropriate to use moxa or laser, which I would usually only use when I want to tonify.

Adeba is a great example of how, as pediatric practitioners, we need to become comfortable with doing very little even when we are working with teenagers. Had I tried to push more treatment onto Adeba, I believe I would have immediately lost his trust. This was a case when the right thing to do was to treat very gently and with a very low dose.

Progression

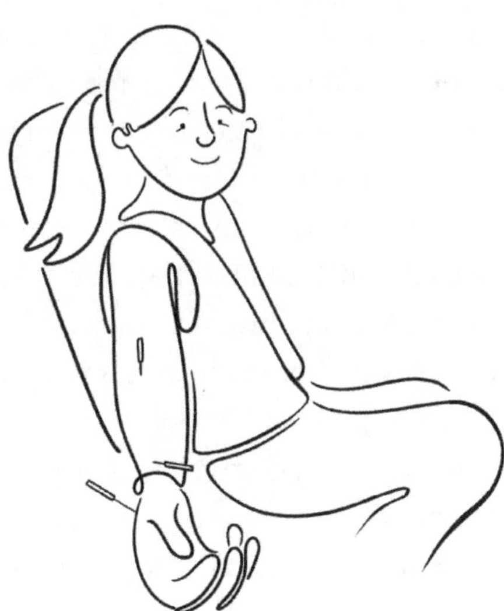

Adeba responded well to his minimal treatment. I felt that the therapeutic relationship we developed was as important as the treatment I gave him. At times, I would feel like I "should" be doing more, but this was a great lesson for me to go at the pace of the young person and to see how, even in the older age groups, we can achieve a lot with such minimal interventions.

Isla—11-year-old with anxiety

Modalities used in clinic: moxibustion; *gua sha*; needles; seeds

Diagnosis: Water constitutional imbalance; Kidney *yin* deficiency; full heat in the Heart

A typical treatment

- Initially, the only modality I used was indirect moxa.
- In time, I added in *gua sha* and seeds.
- After six sessions, Isla readily accepted needles.

Rationale

When Isla arrived for her first treatment, she was so fearful and anxious that she would not even let me take her pulse. She remained on the beanbag, and I sat at her level and chatted to her. Once I had discovered she adored horse riding, she began to relax slightly. It was a hot day, and she was wearing flip flops. She agreed to take them off, and I felt her feet, which were freezing cold. I demonstrated using indirect moxa on her dad, and she agreed that I could try it on her feet (on Ki 1 *yongquan*) as she sat on the beanbag.

Isla had a very strong and positive reaction even to just a little indirect moxa. That meant that next time she came, she was much less nervous. She still wanted to stay on the beanbag and have her treatment fully clothed. I knew I needed to find a way to clear some heat from her Heart. She did not like the idea of any kind of sticker anywhere on her body. So I did some *gua sha* on the Heart channel to vent some heat, as well as some more moxa.

Progression

By treatment three, Isla had let me put some seeds on a couple of ear points. By treatment four, she was a convert to acupuncture! She actually asked me if she could try a needle. Ever since then, she has been happy to be needled anywhere and absolutely loves her treatments. She came a long way in a short period of time from that first treatment.

Summary

My hope is that the cases above help to illustrate that much of the skill involved in being a pediatric acupuncturist comes from being able to think on your feet. We need to bring creativity and adaptability to how we approach treating every child that we see. I also hope that these cases illustrate the importance of prioritizing the therapeutic relationship and learning to go at the child's pace.

Chapter 10

Building and Running a Successful Pediatric Clinic

This chapter will explain clearly the practicalities of an acupuncture appointment for a child. The set-up of our clinic spaces, the timings of our sessions and how we take a case history all need to be considered. Our approach needs to be considerably different than when we are treating adults.

People feng shui

It matters where people sit. Seating arrangements communicate a lot of information. If you go to your sister's wedding, you probably are not going to feel good if you are seated on Table 10, which happens to be the furthest away from the bride and groom. How do you feel if there is a wide table between you and your doctor? Getting the seating right is important.

Good seating arrangements:

- promote good communication
- help a child to feel recognized, respected and important
- help everyone to feel relaxed.

Here are a few key points to think about when planning seating in your clinic:

- Invest in a beanbag. Toddlers and young kids immediately relax when sitting on something squidgy. They can move their body to a position that feels good to them. The degree of "sinking" that happens when you sit on a beanbag means the child feels contained and safe. Even better, invest in two beanbags if you have the space. That way you can sit on one and be at the same level as the child.

- Ensure that your chair, and the chair an older child or teenager sits in, are the same height. You do not want to be looking down on the young person sitting opposite you.

- Have a fold-up chair that you can move around for a parent as needed. With an older child or teenager, I usually place the parent to the side of me so that it's clear the main communication is between me and the young person. If I need to bring the parent in, then I can turn to the side to invite them to answer a question or give their perspective. With a less confident child who wants their parent next to them, I can move the fold-up chair beside their chair or beanbag.

- It's great if your chair has wheels. That way, you can move around easily as you need to. A young person might feel more relaxed if there is a little more space than usual between you and them. If you are going to treat a little one on their parent's lap, you can just seamlessly wheel in closer to them.

Carrying out the treatment: location, location, location...

Finding the best place to carry out your treatment will help determine the degree to which a child will accept your treatment. We adults have often become immune to feeling uncomfortable. We hope that children have not got to that point yet. Where they are, and how they are positioned, really does make a whole lot of difference to how they feel.

Different children will feel comfortable with different set-ups. Some children are comfortable with front-to-front, face-to-face contact. For others, that may feel too direct. These children may prefer that you approach them from the side, where they have the option to turn towards or away from you in order to protect their boundaries. Others feel nervous when anybody is behind them, and this must be taken into account when we are carrying out the treatment.

Here are some of the places children have been as I have carried out their treatments:

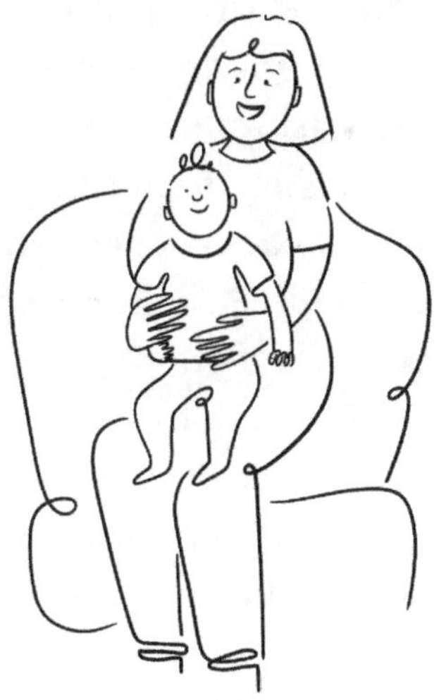

- On the treatment table
- On their parent's lap
- On a beanbag
- On my lap
- Under my treatment table
- Under my desk
- Crawling or running around my entire clinic building
- Outside in the garden.

Be flexible! The only thing that really matters is that the child is comfortable. This is not to say that there aren't times when boundaries need to be set. If we know that a child is quite happy on the treatment table and we can give them a better treatment there, then we may let them know that is where they need to be. We can encourage when there is a slight reluctance but should not insist when there is fear.

Let's walk through an initial session step by step

There are many different ways of creating an initial session so that the young person and their parent feel good at the end of it. I am not an artist, but nevertheless, I think of the process in a way I imagine an artist does when embarking on a painting. I need to be in the right headspace, get into the zone and respond in the moment to what goes on whilst at the same time making sure I keep hold of a vision of what I want the end result to be.

The way I do it will be different to the way you should do it. As we read in the *Zhuangzi*, "He who is not essentially sincere is unable to touch others."[42] So I encourage you to use everything that follows as a guide but also to make it your own.

Step 1—putting everybody at ease

The majority of young people and their parents will feel at the very least a sense of trepidation on their first visit. They don't know what to expect, what you are going to be like or what is going to be involved, and oftentimes they regard you as their final hope. So doing everything you can to make them feel comfortable is a priority. I usually spend the first five to ten minutes simply trying to connect human to human, to put everyone at ease. This may involve chatting about their journey here or asking the child to tell me about the toy they have brought with them or about what they have been doing that day.

Step 2—finding out who the child is

As I discussed in Chapter 2, put your focus initially on finding out *who* the young person is rather than *how* they are. Start with the person, and then gradually move to the symptoms. I may begin with phrases such as, "Tell me a little bit about yourself," or, "What do you love doing the most when you aren't at school?" or, "Who lives in your house with you?"

Step 3—setting the stage for questioning the symptoms and systems

Before I embark on questioning the child's symptoms and systems, I usually say something like, "I am going to ask quite a few questions so I can understand how to help you. I don't mind who answers them—you can answer them all yourself, or Mum/Dad can answer for you if it feels difficult." I usually try to keep things light by also saying, "And you are allowed to disagree with anything that Mum/Dad says too." If I sense that this part of the appointment is going to be difficult for the child, I may also let them know they can tell me at any point if they feel the questions are too much. Or I will automatically cut short the questioning myself if I sense they are struggling. Even if I do not have all the information I want, I can always fill in the gaps at a later stage.

Step 4—preparing the child for treatment

When I have finished questioning, I then explain to the child (in an age-appropriate way) what I would like to do next. So I talk them through how I will take their pulse, look at their tummy, feel their abdomen, etc. Children really like to know what is coming next. After I have finished my palpatory diagnosis, I then let the child know how I would like to deliver their treatment. At every stage, I prepare them for what is coming next, always being sure to give them the option of saying no to something that they are concerned about.

When a child does say no to something, I judge whether or not it feels like a definite no or whether it might be worth demonstrating or explaining more about what I was proposing. There is a fine line between encouragement and coercion.

When working with a baby, instead of preparing them for the treatment, I prepare the parent for the treatment. The parent is the child's voice, so they need to know what is coming next both in order to reassure them and so they can say no to anything they do not feel comfortable with their baby having.

Step 5—carrying out the treatment

There are so many different ways to carry out a treatment on a child, and which one we choose is dependent on the child's nature and state of mind in that moment. Some children like to lie still quietly while they have their treatment. Others like to chat. Some like to read a book or play with a toy. Others like to be very involved in what I am doing. Some will find it easy to stay in the same place for a while, whilst others will find it a challenge. It is easy to deliver your treatment with some children, and it is very challenging with others.

When treating adults, the practitioner's main concern is to cultivate a sense of inner stillness and focus, gather their intention (*yi*) and be fully in the moment. When treating children, we need to do the same. However, at the same time, we also need to "manage" the child, who may be restless, bored, fidgety, defiant or in a very playful mood. Combining these two aspects can be a challenge. There is no "right way" to go about it. There are, however, two guiding principles to bear in mind:

- Stay connected with the child, *shen* to *shen*, as you treat them.
- Summon your intention (*yi*) and your *zhi* (willpower) and make it your goal to complete your treatment!

Please see Chapter 6 for more detailed information on delivering your treatment.

Step 6—post-treatment checking in

When I have finished the child's treatment, I allow some time to talk to them and the parent about how we all feel treatment is going, where we go from here and any questions they may have. This may also be the time when I talk to a parent of a baby or young child about any changes they may be able to make at home that I feel will be helpful for their child.

Step 7—home goals/targets/challenges!

When working with children from around the age of seven or eight onwards, I really like to collaborate with them to set a particular goal. Up until adolescence (when a different approach is needed), I find that the majority of children really love this. It motivates them and helps them to feel empowered. They are often so excited to come back next time and tell me how their "challenge" has gone. Just how we go about this will depend on the nature of the child. Some children are competitive and love having a goal to reach; others need gentle encouragement.

Whatever our approach, what we ask children to do at home is vitally important. It's not simply about excluding something from their diet or spending less time on their screens. It goes deeper than that. It is about finding a way of getting them truly involved in their treatment and teaching them that they can be the architect of their own health.

Ten-year-old Sadie wet the bed every night. Whilst this was rooted in some very clear patterns of imbalance that showed on her tongue and pulse, it was not helped by some of her habits. Sadie never drank anything before or during school, or even when she first got home from school. She consequently loaded all her liquid intake just before bedtime. She also refused to drink water and would only accept fruit squash, which was filled either with sugar or artificial flavors, both of which tend to exacerbate bedwetting. Communication between Sadie and her parents tended to break down over this issue.

Sadie was an Earth-type child. This meant that she easily felt misunderstood. So I started my mission to change her drinking habits by empathizing with her about just how hard it was for her. Earth types tend to respond well when they feel they are *really* understood. They also like to feel someone is *really* looking after them and nurturing them, so I then gave her a special chart I had made where she could fill in each day how she was doing with replacing squash with water and drinking before and during school. Earth types are also often quite conscientious and like to please others, so I made a special effort to show Sadie how happy I was when she came back with her chart and showed me her progress.

I believe that this "homework" was as important as the rest of the treatment. Moreover, it demonstrated to Sadie that her actions could have a positive impact on her health, which is something she could carry forward into her life.

Taking a case history

Generally speaking, taking a history for a child takes less time than it does for an adult simply because they have had fewer years of life. For a young baby, it can take barely any time at all.*

There are a couple of other factors to bear in mind, however. First, you may want to glean some information from the parent before the appointment, especially when there are aspects of the child's health or life that are not appropriate to speak about in front of them. As discussed in Chapter 3, I always have an initial phone call with the parent before booking their child's first appointment. This gives the parent the opportunity to express anything they need to convey out of earshot of the child. Second, when taking the history, give yourself permission to stop when you have the information you need. Filling your head with too many facts, when you already have enough to make an accurate diagnosis, takes you away from feeling the child's *qi*.

* Hub of Pediatric Acupuncture (www.practitioner.pediatricacupuncture.org) members have access to sample intake forms for all ages.

Length of appointment

Although the actual treatment time for a child is short, there are a lot of peripheral aspects which do take time. A child may need to use the toilet, a baby may need a feed or a diaper change and it may take a while for a child to get coats and shoes on and off. Furthermore, you may need some time to chat to the parent, make up an essential oil blend, check in with the child about how they are feeling or discuss what you are encouraging them to do over the week.

I have experimented with different appointment lengths over the years. My aim is to try to find the balance between making my appointments short enough that I can help as many children as possible and long enough that the children get a good treatment and I do not feel rushed or stressed. It's also important for me to have a flow and rhythm to my day, and this can get lost if my appointment slots are too long. It's a fine balance. I encourage you to try things out and find something that feels good for you. As a guide, Table 10.1 illustrates the lengths of my current appointment slots.

Table 10.1 Appointment times for different ages

	Babies and toddlers	Children	Teenagers
Initial session	60 minutes	70 minutes	70 minutes
Follow-up session	30 minutes	35 minutes	40 minutes
Online initial session	60 minutes	60 minutes	60 minutes
Online follow-up	30 minutes	30 minutes	30 minutes

Pricing

I am often asked by practitioners how much they should charge when treating children. There is an unspoken expectation that, because they are little, their treatments should cost less. Of course, how much you charge will depend largely on where you are practicing and what is the norm for your area.

Many practitioners charge for the time they spend treating children relative to how much they charge when treating adults. So if they charge $100 for a one-hour session with an adult, they charge $50 for a 30-minute session with a child. This seems like a fairly sensible way to do things. However, I believe we are charging not only for our time but also for our expertise. If you have done significant postgraduate training in pediatrics, then that makes you a specialist. So you might want to take this into account when deciding on your pricing.

I feel that what is most important is that as a practitioner you feel you are charging enough so as not to feel that you are underselling your expertise and becoming resentful, but not so much that you feel an inordinate amount of pressure to get immediate, outstanding results. The most essential consideration when deciding on your fees is that it feels right for you. You need to make a living but ideally will be able to be flexible in what you charge for families who are under financial strain or for children who will need a lot of ongoing treatment.*

I became frustrated that some children who came to my private clinic were not getting the full benefits of acupuncture because finances prevented them coming as often or for as long as they needed. This was a key reason I set up a low-cost, multibed children's clinic. It feels good to know that I earn enough money in my private practice to pay the bills but also have an option for families that cannot afford private rates.

We all have very different relationships with money. When deciding on what you charge, take a few minutes to reflect to make sure you are not underselling yourself. Acupuncture treatment can change the life trajectory for many, many children. What you offer is of huge value.

---

* I have two clinics. One is my private practice, and one is a low-cost multibed for children. This means I can offer treatment in my multibed to children who really need it and whose families cannot afford the fee in my private practice.

Availability

When treating children, it is necessary to make yourself available at times they will be able to come. In school term times, this will mean having clinics after school and into the early evening, and/or at some point over the weekend.

However, there are a lot of children who can come during the school day. This may be babies and toddlers who aren't yet of school age, children who are too poorly to attend school or home-schooled children. There are also some parents who are prepared to take their child out of school for appointments because they, quite rightly in my opinion, value their child's health over and above their education.

Building up your pediatric practice

In order to attract young people into your clinic. you may need to market yourself slightly differently than you do for your adult practice. Although the tide is changing, there are still many parents who do not know that acupuncture is a treatment that may help their child or that their child would tolerate. Below are a few suggestions.

Tell your adult clients you treat children

Your current adult clients are fertile ground in which to grow your pediatric practice. They are people who already know about and understand some of the benefits possible from acupuncture. Unless you tell them, they may just not know that you can adapt your treatment to children too. Furthermore, you can be sure that most adults who come to see you have either children, grandchildren, nieces or nephews themselves or neighbors, colleagues or friends with children. Put a notice up in your waiting room, make a flyer to give them or, even better, simply talk to them about your treatment of children. It might be a good idea to stress the ways in which your treatment of a child would differ from your treatment of them. Mention the kinds of conditions from which children suffer that you may be able to help with. Crucially, let them know that you can treat children effectively without using needles.

Tell your colleagues you treat children

Let your local acupuncture colleagues, as well as other healthcare professionals such as osteopaths, homeopaths or psychologists, know that you work with children. They may be really happy to know that they can refer people to you. Many of them may not treat children themselves.

Make it clear on your website that you are a specialist

Before a parent brings their child to you, they will want to know that treating children is something you are specifically interested in. In my experience, they will not be so concerned with your specific qualifications but will be reassured by the fact that you regularly see children in your practice and that this is a specialism of yours. Of course, we all have to start somewhere, and some children will necessarily be the first children you ever treat. So if you cannot honestly say you have experience in treating children, then letting people know that this is something you are doing some postgraduate training in will also be reassuring.*

Go to where you are needed

As I write, schools and health services are struggling under the weight of demand. Consequently, huge numbers of children are not getting the support they need, in particular with their mental health. If you can find someone who works in a school or for child mental health services who is open to the idea of acupuncture, they may be relieved to know there is someone they can refer to who may be able to offer support they are struggling to give. Let them know about the evidence for acupuncture in the treatment

---

* For details of postgraduate training in pediatric acupuncture, please go to: https://www.pediatricacupuncture.org/education/.

of anxiety, for example.* There are many children who do not respond well to "talking therapies" for whom acupuncture may be especially useful.

When approaching schools or child mental health services, remember that people who work in these institutions are generally extremely busy and struggling to keep on top of their burgeoning workload. Make it easy for them. Let them know you can be a part of a solution to their problems. You want to avoid creating an extra job for them, so doing as much of the work as possible to set up an easy way for them to refer children to you will increase the chances of this actually happening.

Make connections

In my 25 or so years of practice, I have found the most effective form of marketing to be making meaningful connections with people. If you can talk confidently, articulately and passionately about your work with people you come across, this is more powerful than any paid marketing. It may be that out of every hundred people you talk to, something only directly comes to you from one of them. Yet "the butterfly effect" suggests that small actions can generate large changes in ways which we cannot predict or trace. The more you believe in what you do and communicate that, the more your practice will grow.

Do your best work

It sounds obvious but it needs saying. The best way to build a practice is to do your best work. This does not mean that you need to feel a huge pressure to "cure" every child you see. That is not possible. It means you need to apply yourself and do the very best you can with each child. This incorporates not only the accuracy of your diagnosis and the skill of your treatment but also how you connect with and relate to the child and their

---

* I suggest going to www.evidencebasedacupuncture.org where you will find accessible summaries of available evidence for the treatment of different conditions.

family. I have had referrals from families whose children have not responded especially well to treatment but who feel that I have given them a quality of care and attention that they have not received elsewhere.

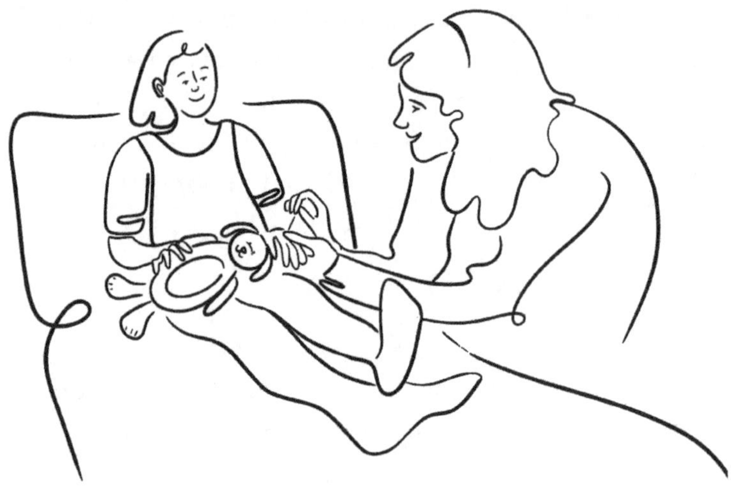

A final word

It is my hope that the information in this chapter will help guide you as you think about creating a clinic where you welcome more young people. I want to balance this by reminding you that perfection is the enemy of the good. There will probably never be a time when you feel you have exactly the right set up, all the knowledge you need and are 100% ready to go. It is in the doing that you will learn, and the only thing to do therefore is to launch yourself into it and enjoy the ride.

Further resources

For all things related to TEAMs pediatrics

Hub of Pediatric Acupuncture (HOPA): https://practitioner.pediatricacupuncture.org

An online community for practitioners working with or interested in working with children, full of support, education, inspiration and a directory of practitioners.

Pediatric acupuncture

Books

Avern, R. (2019) *Acupuncture for Babies, Children and Teenagers: Treating Both the Illness and the Child*. London: Singing Dragon.

Scott, J. and Barlow, T. (1999) *Acupuncture in the Treatment of Children*. Hove: Chinese Medicine Publications.

Courses

TCM Academy of Integrative Medicine: www.tcm.ac/complete-acupuncture-paediatrics

Shonishin

Birch, S. (2011) *Shonishin: Japanese Pediatric Acupuncture*. Stuttgart: Thieme.

Wernicke, T. (2014) *Shonishin: The Art of Non-Invasive Acupuncture*. London: Singing Dragon.

Pediatric *tui na*

Books

Avern, R. (2019) *Acupuncture for Babies, Children and Teenagers: Treating Both the Illness and the Child.* London: Singing Dragon.

Flaws, B. (1985) *Turtle Tail and Other Tender Mercies.* Boulder, CO: Blue Poppy Press.

Rossi, E. (2011) *Pediatrics in Chinese Medicine.* Barnet: Donica.

Ya-li, F. (1994) *Chinese Pediatric Massage Therapy.* Boulder, CO: Blue Poppy Press.

Courses

Hub of Pediatric Acupuncture (HOPA): https://practitioner.pediatricacupuncture.org

Essential Oils

Books

Holmes, P. (2014) *Channeling Fragrance: A Clinical Manual for Using Essential Oils in Chinese Medicine.* Santa Rosa, CA: Snow Lotus Press.

Robert, E. (2022) *Chinese Medicine Essential Oils: A Materia Medica and Practical Guide to Their Use.* San Francisco, CA: Inner Palace Press.

Courses

Tiffany Carole: www.tiffanycarole.com

Snow Lotus: www.snowlotus.org

Laser acupuncture

Kreisel, V. and Weber, M. (2012) *Laser Acupuncture.* Starnberg: Fuchtenbusch.

Five Phase approach to children

Avern, R. (2022) *Chinese Medicine for Childhood Anxiety and Depression: A Practical Guide for Practitioners and Parents.* London: Singing Dragon.

Kalbantner-Wernicke, K. and Wray-Fears, B. (2014) *Children at Their Best.* London: Singing Dragon.

Cowan, S. (2012) *Fire Child, Water Child.* Oakland, CA: New Harbinger.

Bibliography

Avern, R. (2019) *Acupuncture for Babies, Children and Teenagers: Treating Both the Illness and the Child.* London: Singing Dragon.

Avern, R. (2022) *Chinese Medicine for Childhood Anxiety and Depression: A Practical Guide for Practitioners and Parents.* London: Singing Dragon.

Hicks, A., Hicks, J. and Mole, P. (2011) *Five Element Constitutional Acupuncture.* Edinburgh: Churchill Livingstone.

Holmes, P. (2014) *Channeling Fragrance: A Clinical Manual for Using Essential Oils in Chinese Medicine.* Santa Rosa, CA: Snow Lotus Press.

Larre, C. (1994) *The Way of Heaven.* Cambridge: Monkey Press.

Larre, C. and Rochat de la Vallée, E. (1995) *Rooted in Spirit.* New York: Station Hill Press.

Rossi, E. (2023) *The Therapeutic Relationship in Acupuncture.* Milan: Network Olistico Internazionale.

Weiger, L. (1965) *Chinese Characters.* New York: Dover Publications.

Wernicke, T. (2014) *Shonishin: The Art of Non-Invasive Acupuncture.* London: Singing Dragon.

Wilms, S. (trans.) (2013) *Venerating the Root: Part 1.* Corbett, OR: Happy Goat Publications.

Wilms, S. (trans.) (2015) *Venerating the Root: Part 2.* Corbett, OR: Happy Goat Publications.

Wilms, S. (trans.) (2022) *Healing Virtue-Power: Medical Ethics and the Doctor's Dao.* Whidbey Island, WA: Happy Goat Productions.

Endnotes

Foreword

1 Sūn Sī Miao *Appended Formulas Worth a Thousand Nuggets of Gold. Beiji Qianjin Yaofang* 備急千金要方.

2 Lo, B., Inn, M., Amacker, R. and Foe, S. (1982) *The Essence of T'ai Chi Ch'uan: The Literary Tradition*. Berkeley CA: North Atlantic Books, p.87.

Chapter 1

3 Wilms, S. (trans.) (2013) *Venerating the Root: Part 1. Sūn Sī Miao's Bei Ji Qian Jin Yao Fang, Volume 5: Pediatrics*. Portland, OR: Happy Goat Productions, p.xviii.

4 Wilms, S. (trans.) (2022) *Healing Virtue-Power: Medical Ethics and the Doctor's Dao*. Whidbey Island, WA: Happy Goat Productions, p.93.

5 Milne, A. A. (2003) *Winnie-the-Pooh*. New York: Harper Children's Audio.

6 Larre, C. and Rochat de la Vallée, E. (1994) *The Way of Heaven*. Cambridge: Monkey Press, p.164.

7 Lu, H. (1972) *A Complete Translation of the Yellow Emperor's Classic of Internal Medicine (Nei Jing and Nan Jing)*. Vancouver: Academy of Oriental Heritage, p.101.

8 Stevenson, R. (dir.) (1964) *Mary Poppins*. Disney. Buena Vista Distribution Company.

9 Larre, C. and Rochat de la Vallée, E. (2001) *The Lung*. Cambridge: Monkey Press, p.54.

10 *Ibid*, p.45.

11 Larre, C. and Rochat de la Vallée, E. (2004) *Spleen and Stomach*. Cambridge: Monkey Press, p.20.

12 Wilms, S. (trans.) and Sūn Sī Miao (2022) *Healing Virtue-Power: Medical Ethics and the Doctor's Dao*. Whidbey Island, WA: Happy Goat Productions, p.17.

13 Larre, C. and Rochat de la Vallée, E. (1995) *Rooted in Spirit: The Heart of Chinese Medicine*. New York: Station Hill Press, p.16.

14 Wilms, S. (trans.) (2022) *Healing Virtue-Power: Medical Ethics and the Doctor's Dao*. Whidbey Island, WA: Happy Goat Productions, p.16.
15 Dylan, B. (2011) "Open the Door, Homer." *The Bootleg Series, Vol. 11: the Basement Tapes Complete, Disc 4*. New York: Columbia.
16 Wilms, S. (trans.) (2022) *Healing Virtue-Power: Medical Ethics and the Doctor's Dao*. Whidbey Island, WA: Happy Goat Productions, p.95.
17 Larre, C. and Rochat de la Vallée, E. (1992) *The Secret Treatise of the Spiritual Orchid*. Cambridge: Monkey Press, p.53.
18 Kipling, R. (1910) *Rewards and Fairies*. Macmillan and Co: London. pp.181–182.
19 Wilms, S. (trans.) (2022) *Healing Virtue-Power: Medical Ethics and the Doctor's Dao*. Whidbey Island, WA: Happy Goat Productions, p.111.

Chapter 2

20 Colman, A. (2008) *A Dictionary of Psychology*. Oxford University Press. www.oxfordreference.com/display/10.1093/oi/authority.20110803100404600
21 Weiger, L. (1965) *Chinese Characters: Their Origin, Etymology, History, Classification and Signification*. New York: Dover Publications, p.641.
22 Rossi, E. (2023) *The Therapeutic Relationship in Acupuncture*. Milan: Network Olistico Internazionale, p.6.
23 Quoted in Hicks, A., Hicks, J. and Mole, P. (2011) *Five Element Constitutional Acupuncture*. Edinburgh: Churchill Livingstone, p.36.
24 Wilms, S. (trans.) (2022) *Healing Virtue-Power: Medical Ethics and the Doctor's Dao*. Whidbey Island, WA: Happy Goat Productions, p.93.
25 Quoted in Hicks, A., Hicks, J. and Mole, P. (2011) *Five Element Constitutional Acupuncture*. Edinburgh: Churchill Livingstone, p.37.
26 Merton, T. (trans.) (1970) *The Way of Chuang Tzu*. London: George Allen and Unwin, pp.75–76.
27 Peabody, F. W. (1984) 'Landmark article March 19, 1927: The care of the patient. By Francis W. Peabody.' *JAMA 252*, 6, 813–818.

Chapter 4

28 Needham, J. (1956) *Science and Civilisation in China, Volume 2*. Cambridge: Cambridge University Press, p.55.
29 Zuozhi, L. and Wilms, S. (trans.) (2014) *Let the Radiant Yang Shine Forth: Lectures on Virtue by Liu Yousheng*. Corbett, OR: Happy Goat Productions. p.66.
30 Maté, G. (2000) *Scattered: How Attention Deficit Disorder Originates and What You Can Do About It*. New York: Plume Printing, p.55
31 Sunu, K. (1985) *The Canon of Acupuncture*. Los Angeles, CA: Yuin University Press, p.85.
32 Richter, F. (2024) The rising prevalence of autism. Autism and Developmental

Disabilities Monitoring Network CDC. www.statista.com/chart/29630/identified-prevalence-of-autism-spectrum-disorder-in-the-us

33 Quoted in Hicks, A., Hicks, J. and Mole, P. (2011) *Five Element Constitutional Acupuncture*. Edinburgh: Churchill Livingstone, p.36.

34 Wilms, S. (trans.) (2024) *Healing Virtue-Power: Medical Ethics and the Doctor's Dao*. Whidbey Island, WA: Happy Goat Productions, p.129.

Chapter 6

35 Wilms, S. (2013) *Venerating the Root: Part 1. Sūn Sī Miao's Bei Ji Qian Jin Yao Fang, Volume 5: Paediatrics*. Portland, OR: Happy Goat Productions, p.123.

36 Quoted in Rossi, E. (2023) *The Therapeutic Relationship in Acupuncture*. Milan: Network Olistico Internazionale, p.xxxiii.

37 Wilms, S. (trans.) (2022) *Healing Virtue-Power: Medical Ethics and the Doctor's Dao*. Whidbey Island, WA: Happy Goat Productions, p.17.

38 Yang, S.-Z. and Chace, C. (trans.) (1994) *Huang Fu Mi: The Systematic Classic of Acupuncture and Moxibustion*. Boulder, CO: Blue Poppy Press, p.181.

39 Zhen, J. (1996) *Da Cheng*. Hong Kong: Guang Publishing Company, p.158.

40 Quoted in Solomon, A. (2016) 'Literature about medicine may be all that can save us.' *The Guardian*. www.theguardian.com/books/2016/apr/22/literature-about-medicine-may-be-all-that-can-save-us

Chapter 8

41 Holmes, P. (2014) *Channeling Fragrance: A Clinical Manual for Using Essential Oils in Chinese Medicine*. Santa Rosa, CA: Snow Lotus Press, p.8.

Chapter 10

42 Quoted in Rossi, E. (2023) *The Therapeutic Relationship in Acupuncture*. Milan: Network Olistico Internazionale, p.6.

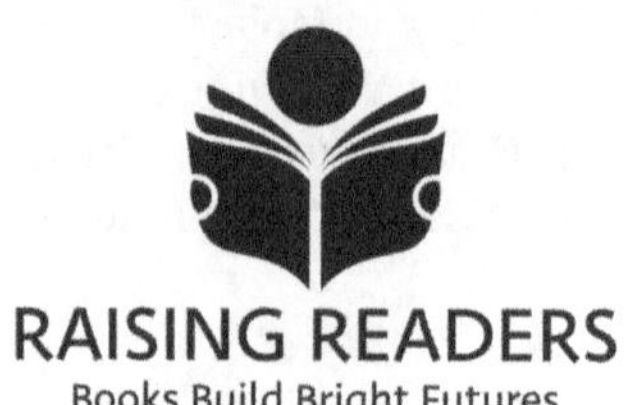

Dear Reader,

We'd love your attention for one more page to tell you about the crisis in children's reading, and what we can all do.

Studies have shown that reading for fun is the **single biggest predictor of a child's future life chances** – more than family circumstance, parents' educational background or income. It improves academic results, mental health, wealth, communication skills, ambition and happiness.[1]

The number of children reading for fun is in rapid decline. Young people have a lot of competition for their time. In 2024, 1 in 10 children and young people in the UK aged 5 to 18 did not own a single book at home.[2]

Hachette works extensively with schools, libraries and literacy charities, but here are some ways we can all raise more readers:

- Reading to children for just 10 minutes a day makes a difference
- Don't give up if children aren't regular readers – there will be books for them!
- Visit bookshops and libraries to get recommendations
- Encourage them to listen to audiobooks
- Support school libraries
- Give books as gifts

There's a lot more information about how to encourage children to read on our website: **www.RaisingReaders.co.uk**

Thank you for reading.

hachette UK

1 OECD, '21st-Century Readers: Developing Literacy Skills in a Digital World', 2021, https://www.oecd.org/en/publications/21st-century-readers_a83d84cb-en.html

2 National Literacy Trust, 'Book Ownership in 2024', November 2024, https://literacytrust.org.uk/research-services/research-reports/book-ownership-in-2024